SURGERY CLERKSHIP

150 BIGGEST
MISTAKES

AND HOW TO
AVOID THEM

CLERKSHIP MISTAKE SERIES

SURGERY CLERKSHIP

150 BIGGEST MISTAKES
AND HOW TO
AVOID THEM

EDITED BY Samir P. Desai, M.D.

AUTHORED BY Samir P. Desai, M.D. • Neal Barshes, M.D.
Ajay Maker, M.D. • Vairavan Subramanian, M.D. • Abhay Bilolikar, M.D.
Alpen Patel, M.D. • Shawn P. Fagan, M.D. • Charles F. Bellows, M.D.

PUBLISHED BY

MD2B

HOUSTON, TEXAS
www.MD2B.net

The Surgery Clerkship: 150 Biggest Mistakes and How to Avoid Them is published by MD2B, P.O. Box 300988, Houston, Texas 77230-0988.

www.MD2B.net

NOTICE: The author and publisher disclaim any personal liability, either directly or indirectly, for advice or information presented within. The author and publisher have used care and diligence in the preparation of this book. Every effort has been made to ensure the accuracy and completeness of information contained within this book. The reader should understand, however, that most of the subject matter of the book is not rooted in scientific observation. The recommendations made within this book have come from the authors' personal experiences and interactions with other attending physicians, residents, and students over many years. Since expectations vary from medical school to medical school, clerkship to clerkship, and resident to resident, the recommendations are not universally applicable. No responsibility is assumed for errors, inaccuracies, omissions, or any false or misleading implication that may arise due to the text.

Printed in the United States of America

ISBN # 0-9725561-3-3

Contents

Chapter 3: Preoperative Note

Chapter 4: Brief Operative Note

Chapter 5: Postoperative Note

Chapter 6: Daily Progress Note

Chapter 7: Operating Room

Chapter 8: Attending Interactions

Chapter 9: On Call

Chapter 10: Surgical Oral Examination

Chapter 11: Studying for the Written Examination

About the Editor

Samir P. Desai, M.D.

Dr. Samir Desai serves on the faculty of the Baylor College of Medicine in the Department of Medicine. Dr. Desai has educated and mentored both medical students and residents, work for which he has received teaching awards. He is an author and editor, having written ten books that together have sold over 70,000 copies worldwide.

Dr. Desai is the author of the popular *101 Biggest Mistakes 3rd Year Medical Students Make and How to Avoid Them*, a book that has helped students reach their full potential during the third year of medical school. In the book, *The Residency Match: 101 Biggest Mistakes and How to Avoid Them*, Dr. Desai shows applicants how to avoid commonly made mistakes during the residency application process. He is also the editor of the Clerkship MIstakes Series, a series of books developed to help students perform at a high level during clinical rotations and acquire the skills needed for a successful career as a physician.

Dr. Desai conceived and authored the Clinician's Guide Series, a series of books dedicated to providing clinicians with practical approaches to commonly encountered problems. Now in its third edition, the initial book in this series, the *Clinician's Guide to Laboratory Medicine*, has become a popular book for third-year medical students, providing a step-by-step approach to laboratory test interpretation. Other titles in this series include the *Clinician's Guide to Diagnosis* and *Clinician's Guide to Internal Medicine*.

In 2002, he founded www.md2b.net, a website committed to helping today's medical student becomes tomorrow's doctor. At the site, a variety of tools and resources are available to help students tackle the challenges of medical school.

After completing his residency training in Internal Medicine at Northwestern University in Chicago, Illinois, Dr. Desai had the opportunity of serving as chief medical resident. He received his MD degree from Wayne State University School of Medicine in Detroit, Michigan, graduating first in his class.

About the Authors

Neal Barshes, M.D.

Dr. Neal R. Barshes graduated *magna cum laude* with a degree in psychology from the University of Illinois in Urbana and then graduated Alpha Omega Alpha from the College of Medicine at the University of Illinois in Chicago. He is currently completing his general surgery residency at the Michael E. DeBakey Department of Surgery at the Baylor College of Medicine in Houston, Texas. During his first year at this program he was selected "Intern of the Year" by faculty and fellow residents. Upon completion of his general surgery residency training, Dr. Barshes will complete fellowship training in solid organ transplant surgery and pursue a career in academic surgery.

Ajay Maker, M.D.

Dr. Ajay Maker graduated from Brown University with honors degrees in Fine Art and Biology, and obtained his medical degree with honors from Yale University School of Medicine in New Haven, Connecticut. He is a general surgery resident at Brigham and Women's Hospital in Boston, Massachusetts, and is currently doing a surgical oncology fellowship with the National Cancer Institute at the NIH in Bethesda, Maryland. He is very interested in medical student education, is the recipient of an Excellence in Teaching residency award, and has authored chapters on clinical medical student education.

Vairavan Subramanian, M.D.

Dr. Vairavan Subramanian graduated *cum laude* from Yale University in 2001 with a Bachelor of Science in Molecular, Cellular, and Developmental Biology. Originally from Houston, he returned to his home town for medical school at the Baylor College of Medicine. His interest in medical education and teaching at all levels led him to pursue a national board position in the American Association of Medical Colleges' Organization of Student Representatives where he helped guide medical school curricula at a national level. In June 2005 he will begin his residency in urologic surgery at the Cleveland Clinic in Ohio.

Abhay Bilolikar, M.D.

Abhay Bilolikar is originally from Troy, Michigan and attended college at Wayne State University in Detroit, Michigan where he received the Bachelor of Science degree in Biology, graduating *summa cum laude* in 2000. He obtained his medical degree from the Wayne State University School of Medicine in 2005. In June 2005, he will begin his residency in Internal Medicine at the University of Michigan in Ann Arbor, Michigan. Over the years, he has enjoyed teaching and tutoring and wishes to do more of the same in the future as a resident and physician.

Alpen Patel, M.D.

Dr. Alpen Patel is an Assistant Professor in the Division of Otolaryngology at the George Washington University School of Medicine. He is also the Director of Rhinology & Allergy. Dr. Patel has educated and mentored many medical students & residents. Dr. Patel received his M.D. degree from the Baylor College of Medicine, graduating with honors. Afterwards, he attended the University of Minnesota, where he completed his residency and obtained a Master's degree in Otolaryngology.

Shawn P. Fagan, M.D.

Dr. Shawn Fagan is an Assistant Professor of Surgery in the Michael E. DeBakey Department of Surgery in Houston, Texas. He received his medical degree and general surgery training at the Baylor College of Medicine. He is currently a staff physician at the Michael E. DeBakey Veterans Affairs Medical Center in Houston, Texas.

Charles F. Bellows, M.D.

Dr. Charles Bellows is an Assistant Professor of Surgery in the Michael E. DeBakey Department of Surgery at the Baylor College of Medicine in Houston, Texas. He is also the Chief of Laparoscopic Surgery at the Michael E. DeBakey Veterans Affairs Medical Center. He received his medical degree from the Medical College of Pennsylvania in Philadelphia. He completed a residency in general surgery at Tulane University in New Orleans.

Foreword

The sheer volume of information that must be absorbed and retained by medical students during their surgery clerkship is only outdone by the short amount of time in which it must be accomplished.

In such a hurried and hectic environment of early-morning rounds, presenting patients, the writing of operative notes and being responsible for a breadth of patient information, it is not surprising that mistakes will occur. However, although an unwelcome component of the learning process, mistakes often prove to be the most poignant tool of learning, providing an opportunity for correction and instruction in proper technique and procedure.

This new book, titled the *Surgery Clerkship: 150 Biggest Mistakes and How to Avoid Them*, is an indispensable tool for guiding the medical student through a tough and challenging clerkship by identifying commonly-made errors and providing plans of action for avoiding them. One such plan suggests students prepare and carry with them templates outlining the types of information required for certain tasks such as the writing of pre and post-operative notes.

Preparation is the key to successfully completing the surgical clerkship. Because students' performance during clerkship is heavily evaluated, and if poor can lead to unsatisfactory opinions that can follow them beyond medical school, it is imperative that students enter into this phase of training as equipped as possible and aware of the expectations that will be placed on them by interns, residents and attending physicians. This new book will not only prepare the student for the tasks and responsibilities of surgical clerkship, but will provide a head start that is sure to impress.

Experience is the name everyone gives to their mistakes. —Oscar Wilde **(1854 - 1900)**, *Lady Windermere's Fan, 1892, Act III*

F. Charles Brunicardi, M.D., F.A.C.S.
DeBakey/Bard Professor and Chairman
Michael E. DeBakey Department of Surgery
Baylor College of Medicine
Houston, Texas

Preface

Your surgery rotation promises to be one of the most challenging rotations you will take during your clinical years of medical school. Over a two or three-month period, you will be expected to master a tremendous amount of information and learn how to diagnose and manage patients with surgical disease. To reach these goals, you will have a plethora of books from which to choose.

In writing this book, our goal was not to duplicate the efforts of other authors, who have written books focusing on the diagnosis and management of patients with surgical disease. Instead, our aim is to provide you with the detailed knowledge you need to function at an intern level. To function at an intern level, you not only need to know about your patient's illness but you also need to know how to perform the tasks involved in the care of your patient. In other words, you need to know how to preround, present patients during work rounds, write surgical notes, handle yourself in the operating room, interact with the attending, and fulfill your responsibilities on call. This book will give you explicit instructions on how to perform these tasks well—not at a student level but at an intern level.

We strive to help you reach this level sooner rather than later by informing you of the major mistakes that students make during the clerkship. By the end of the rotation, most students learn to avoid these mistakes through a process of trial and error. Wouldn't it be better, though, if you could avoid these mistakes altogether? With this book, you can and armed with this knowledge, you will speed up your learning curve, reduce your anxiety level, and quickly reach a comfort level that allows you to do your best work. We wish you the best during the surgery clerkship and hope that this book becomes your companion, providing you with the tools needed to tackle the challenges of this rotation.

—Samir Desai, M.D.

Prerounds

During the surgery clerkship your day will typically begin with prerounds. During prerounds you will see your patients alone. The goal is to identify any new events that have occurred in your patient's course after you left the hospital on the previous day. The information that you gather will be presented to the residents and interns during work rounds, which immediately follow prerounds. In this chapter we will discuss commonly made mistakes during prerounds.

Mistake **#1**

Setting aside too little time for prerounds

It is important that you set aside sufficient time for prerounding. When you are short on time, the quality of your work is likely to suffer. This will certainly be apparent to your resident and intern during work rounds when you are asked to present your patients to the team.

The amount of time that should be allotted for prerounds depends on a number of factors. The answers to the following questions will help you determine the time needed.

● **What are your responsibilities during prerounds?**

   In general, students are expected to gather important patient data (see Mistake # 2), analyze the information, and be ready to present this information to the team during work rounds.

1

- **Do you have to write daily progress notes during prerounds?**

  At most institutions, students are asked to write daily progress notes during prerounds. If you are at an institution that has adopted this practice, you will have to set aside time during prerounds for the writing of these notes.

- **Is it early or late in the rotation?**

  If you have done other rotations, you know how difficult it is to operate at peak efficiency early in the rotation. During the first week or so, the newness of the environment and unfamiliarity with expectations create a situation in which tasks are completed more slowly. With time, your comfort level rises and routines are established, both of which increase efficiency and pare down the amount of time you require for prerounds.

- **How many patients are you following?**

  It stands to reason that the time needed for prerounds will increase as the number of patients you are following rises.

- **How complicated or sick are your patients?**

  Obviously, hospitalized patients are sick. But there are different degrees of sickness. Patients in the surgical intensive care unit, for example, often have multiple problems. These patients are seriously ill, and your assessment of their condition will naturally take longer.

Answering these questions before you call it a night will help you determine what time you should arrive for prerounds the following day. Your goal should be to complete your prerounding with time to spare. In the event that a task takes longer than expected, this extra cushion of time will come in quite handy. The time that is left can also be used to polish your presentation for work rounds. Your presentations on work rounds are your time to display your progress and skills. It is evident during a presentation who took the time to gather information and talk to their patient, and who rushed through the morning.

Success Tip #1

Daily progress notes usually need to be completed before work rounds begin. Make sure you leave enough time for note writing.

Success Tip #2

Give yourself extra time to see patients in the ICU.

Mistake #2

Incomplete data gathering during prerounds

A considerable amount of patient data needs to be gathered during prerounds. This information will allow you to make an assessment of the patient's condition and decide on the day's plan. You will present your findings and thoughts to the rest of the team during work rounds. In addition, the information will form a large part of that day's progress note. Following is a checklist that you can use to make sure you have gathered the necessary data.

Checklist for prerounds

- ☐ Postoperative day # (if applicable)
- ☐ Vital signs (T_{max}, $T_{current}$, RR, BP, P)
- ☐ Ins/Outs (24 hour & morning shift)
- ☐ List of current medications
- ☐ Antibiotic therapy (name and day of therapy)
- ☐ Patient's complaints/concerns
- ☐ Physical examination
- ☐ Events overnight according to nurse
- ☐ New notes in the chart
- ☐ New lab test results
- ☐ New microbiology test results
- ☐ New imaging test results
- ☐ New orders since you last saw the patient

With time, most students become quite comfortable gathering information during prerounds. It is more difficult to take the information that is gathered, analyze it, and then use it to formulate the patient's management plan for the day. At the student level, it is not easy to formulate the plan, but many students do not even make an attempt to do so. During work rounds, these students simply present the information and wait for the resident to outline the plan for the day, which they will then help execute.

It is important to realize that star students will do more than just gather information during prerounds. They will set aside time before work rounds to review the information, understand its clinical significance, and use it to formulate the plan for the day.

Success Tip #3

The star student not only gathers the necessary data but also sets time aside to organize and process the information before presenting the patient to the team during work rounds.

4

Mistake **#3**

Information gathered during prerounds is not written down

Keep an organized system of data gathering that you can use to refer to before or during your morning presentation. Write down the objective information you gathered on prerounds in the order that you will present it. Keep this reference and add to it daily. For example, each new entry on your patient reference can have a line: "POD #__, Abx__/day#__, T_{max}, $T_{current}$, HR, BP, RR, O_2 sat, O_2 amount, Ins/Outs: PO, IVF, urine output, miscellaneous output, new labs, new microbiology results, new radiography." If you don't write it down, you will forget it.

Mistake **#4**

Not being intimately familiar with the patient's chart

The medical chart is the record of the patient's hospital course. It is the main form of communication between the various teams, consultants, and allied health professionals, especially since most other caregivers visit the patient and read the chart when the surgery team is in the OR.

To be an excellent medical student, you should be intimately familiar with your patient's chart. Because information will have been added to the chart while you were away, it is useful to begin prerounds by reading the patient's chart. After looking over the notes and orders written by nurses, covering house staff, and consultants, you will quickly be brought up to speed on your patient's hospital course. Of course, you will also want to check the chart often throughout the day to look for updates—notes from consulting services, nurses, results, etc. Know what information to take special note of—for example, if your team is awaiting consultation from the infectious disease service—you should be checking the chart often for their recommendations.

Surgical progress notes are notoriously illegible and brief. Sometimes orders that are written by your resident or the covering resident may not be clearly documented in the progress note. That's why it's always important to look at the orders during prerounds. If you don't do so, you run the risk of missing some important information. As an example, let's say your 72-year old patient had difficulty falling asleep. The covering resident wrote an order for Benadryl but did not document this in the progress note. During prerounds, your patient is confused. As you consider potential causes, you do not consider Benadryl as an etiology because you are not aware that it was ordered. In work rounds, you are informed that the confusion is likely due to the Benadryl given to the patient during the night. You will avoid this situation if you habitually look over the orders during prerounds.

Success Tip #4
Strive to function as the intern for every patient you are following.

Mistake #5

Not tracking down lab or examination results

Sometimes a test is ordered, but the results are not available at the typical time. The residents will consider you a valuable member of the team if you discover why the results are not available.

Typically this involves tracing the steps of the test or examination in question. After a lab test order is written, it is read by the nurse. Blood may be drawn by a nurse or a phlebotomist, and then taken to the lab. The lab then performs the test and makes the results available in some fashion (hard copy, computer record, etc.). So, retrace these steps: Was the order written? Was the order noted by the nurses? Was the blood drawn? Did the lab receive the blood?

Mistake **#6**

Not offering to help your residents preround on patients even if they're not your own

Surgical residents typically carry a heavy patient load but have few precious hours in the morning to see them. Offering to help with patients you are not following will win you major points and make residents more interested in teaching you during free moments. Residents appreciate when students volunteer to look up vital signs for the team, change dressings, pull drain tubes, remove staples, gather radiology films, etc.

Success Tip #5

Efforts to ease the heavy workload on your interns and residents will be greatly appreciated. Your rewards may include additional teaching and opportunities to perform procedures.

Success Tip #6

The best evaluations are often given to students who help out whenever and wherever assistance is needed.

Mistake #7

Not knowing which patients you will see in the morning

Before you check out for the day, ask your intern and the other students on your team who will see which patients in the morning. Surgical prerounds typically start very early in the morning and are fast paced. The last thing you want to do is page your intern at 5 a.m. because you don't know which patients you're supposed to round on. The shortened work hours are changing the way rounds are done but you will still see your patient(s) before work rounds. It is a vital part of your education and the best way to establish rapport with your patient.

Mistake #8

Being short with the ancillary staff

As you race to complete prerounds, members of the ancillary staff may approach you to discuss some aspect of your patient's care. The last thing you may want is to be slowed down. After all, there's much that needs to be done before work rounds begin. It is important, however, to take the time to listen to their concerns or questions. They may have information that is vital to your prerounding. They can also help you locate supplies and facilitate the completion of tasks, increasing your efficiency.

In their haste to complete their prerounding, students have been known to be short with staff or even rude. Remember that rude or unpleasant behavior is not forgotten, and there simply is no excuse for it. An entire team of caregivers is needed to provide exceptional patient care.

Success Tip #7

Pay attention to concerns or issues raised by members of the ancillary staff (e.g., nurses). Read their notes carefully. Their input is valuable for optimal patient care.

Success Tip #8

Treat everyone with respect.

Mistake **#9**

Spending little or no time talking with the patient

It might seem obvious to talk to a patient during prerounds. However, when you are hectically prerounding at 5:15 a.m. in a dark patient room, you may wonder whether you should wake the patient. Do not enter a room and begin examining a patient or taking down their dressing without first politely waking the patient and introducing yourself. Do respect wishes to be left undisturbed. Furthermore, always ask a patient how they are feeling, if there are any changes in their pain, or if they have particular concerns or questions for the team.

Sometimes students are singularly focused on the pursuit of objective information (vital signs, lab test results) to such an extent that little or no discussion takes place between the student and the patient. When this happens, patients feel that their concerns are not being addressed and this can damage the rapport and trust that you have established with the patient. It is also important to understand that the objective information should always be evaluated and interpreted in the context of how the patient feels. That's difficult to do if you're not spending enough time talking with them.

Mistake #10

Not examining the patient thoroughly

ALWAYS examine the patient. Your morning examination is the best assessment of overnight events and is the first defense against untoward events. It is helpful to think of the patient by "systems." The following is a comprehensive systems approach to the morning physical examination. It is a directed examination to be used as a guide for the generic surgical patient. Obviously, some patients may have specific concerns you should pay attention to. The morning examination should take five minutes or less. Practice to do this efficiently, not only for the patient's pre-dawn comfort, but also to decrease the time you need to preround.

● **Neurologic**

Talk to the patient while you are examining them and establish alertness and orientation. Ask them if they have any nausea or headaches and observe their pupils, eye movements, speech, and posture.

● **Cardiac**

Listen to the patient's heart. Is there a new murmur? Is the patient's heart rhythm regular or irregular?

Often, in non-telemetry patients, auscultation of an irregularly, irregular heart rhythm is the first indication of atrial fibrillation, a common problem in certain postoperative patient populations.

● **Pulmonary**

Listen to all lung zones with the patient sitting up. Pay special attention for signs of progressive atelectasis or pneumonia.

● **Gastrointestinal**

Ask the patient if he or she has passed gas and when his or her last bowel movement was (they are not always recorded correctly). While palpating the abdomen, pay special attention to the presence of tympany or distention. Listen for the presence or absence of bowel sounds.

● **Genitourinary**

Examine the Foley for patency and condition. Take note of the color and character of the urine.

● **Hematology**

Assess the legs for symmetry, tenderness, swelling, and other signs of DVT. Palpate distal pulses. If you are unable to palpate a pulse, use a Doppler device.

● **Infectious Disease**

Assess all venipuncture, drain, and line sites for evidence of infection. Check the wound for cleanliness, healing progress, and evidence of infection (i.e., smell and presence of discharge).

Mistake **#11**

Withholding patient information from the intern or resident

Students sometimes withhold patient information, thinking that they will look good if they know something their intern or resident does not. They wait for that perfect opportunity when the passing of the information will put them in the best possible light with the senior resident or attending physician. These students fail to recognize that this practice is certainly not in the best interest of the patient. The way to excel is to know everything there is to know about your patient and to relay pertinent information up the chain of command.

While a medical student might look bad if a resident or intern knows something about the patient that he or she does not, the converse is not true. You will earn respect and trust by informing your intern of any important information you gained on prerounds before starting work rounds. Senior residents and attendings can tell who is working hard, and they are looking for people to help the team provide efficient and excellent care, not for anyone to stand out.

Success Tip #9

Always communicate patient information with the team member who is directly above you. If you withhold information until the "right time" in an attempt to make yourself look better, it's likely to backfire.

Success Tip #10

Never lose sight of the fact that you are a member of a team. Do not place your own interests above that of the team. Remember that there is no "I" in team.

Morning Work Rounds

During morning work rounds, the team (usually without the attending physician) travels from room to room, seeing each of the patients on the service. The most junior member of the team (junior medical student, physician assistant student, senior medical student, intern) who is following the patient is required to update the team on the patient's progress. This update will include any significant events that have occurred overnight, the results of any lab/diagnostic testing, and the current condition of the patient. The information you present will help the team formulate a diagnostic and therapeutic plan.

This chapter highlights the main difference between internal medicine and surgery. Rounds, progress notes, orders, test scheduling, and consults are often completed before 7:30 a.m., when most other physicians arrive to the hospital. Patients need to be properly evaluated and treated before the team goes to the OR for the rest of the day. Commonly made mistakes during morning work rounds are discussed in this chapter.

Mistake **#12**

Being unfamiliar with the resident's expectations for you during morning work rounds

With any new job or assignment, it's difficult to do your best work if you are not sure what is expected of you. That's certainly true of the surgery clerkship as well. On the first day of the rotation, it is important to meet with members of the team. They will fill you in on your day-to-day responsibilities, one of which is morning work rounds. After having this discussion, you should have a clear understanding of what happens during work rounds. You should not leave this meeting without having these questions answered.

Questions to ask about morning work rounds

- What time do work rounds start?
- Where do work rounds start?
- How would you like me to present newly admitted patients?
- How would you like me to present established patients?
- What information would you like me to include in these presentations?
- How much time do I have to present the patient?
- Do progress notes need to be completed before work rounds begin?

You will be at your best in work rounds only after you reach a certain comfort level. The first step in reaching that level is to be clear on the team's expectations of you during these rounds. Once you are aware of these expectations, you can do everything in your power to meet their needs.

Mistake **#13**

Arriving late for work rounds

Since all patients on the service need to be seen before going to the OR, and the OR start time is not flexible, there is little tolerance for tardiness. To avoid any problems, show up for work rounds about five minutes before they are set to begin. Make sure your watch is accurate. Of course, you cannot be on time *and* prepared for work rounds unless you have left enough time for prerounds (see Mistake #1).

Success Tip #11
Always be on time for work rounds.

Mistake **#14**

Oral patient presentations are not brief and concise

Repeat after us: Brief and concise. Brief and concise. These are the adjectives that should be used to describe your patient presentations during work rounds. Patient census on the surgery service is often much larger than what you may have been accustomed to on other rotations. All of these patients need to be seen with their daily progress notes and orders written before the first case in the OR begins. Since there is so much to do, the team must operate at peak efficiency. Although there are many ways students can help improve team efficiency, chief among these is delivering brief patient presentations. Presentations on uncomplicated patients should not take more than 45 to 60 seconds.

Success Tip #12

Practice your work rounds presentation at the end of prerounds (before work rounds begin). Make sure that you convey the necessary information in an organized manner without exceeding the allotted time.

Success Tip #13

Aim to present your patients without relying heavily on your notes. You should be able to convey the patient's symptoms and physical examination findings from memory. Lab test and other quantitative data need not be memorized.

Mistake #15

Presenting patients in a disorganized fashion

Giving disorganized patient presentations is perhaps the most common error committed by medical students during work rounds. There is definitely an order to the work rounds presentation and students who adhere to the proper order are clearly seen as being more "with it" then students who do not. Most residents expect that you will use the SOAP format (subjective, objective, assessment, plan) for the work rounds presentation, which is essentially the same order that you will use for writing the patient's daily progress note. Please refer to the list that follows for more information.

Step-by-step approach to the work rounds presentation

Step 1: Start your work rounds presentation with a short summary of the patient to remind the team of his or her problems. Present the patient to the team by giving the patient's name, age, gender, and chief complaint or working diagnosis/reason for being in the hospital. **For the postoperative patient,** also state the postoperative day #, operation, and indication for operation.

Example: This is postoperative day #2 for Mr. Jones, a 72-year old man, s/p left hemicolectomy for colon adenocarcinoma.

Step 2: Present the subjective data, which should include how the patient's symptom(s) have changed, new symptoms, and events that have occurred since yesterday's rounds. For the postoperative patient, also report physical activity, use of incentive spirometer, pain control, and bowel habits.

Example: He has no new complaints. His pain is minimal. He has tolerated sips of clear liquids without difficulty. He said he passed flatus once during the night. He walked around the ward three times yesterday and once earlier this morning.

Step 3: Present the objective data, beginning with the vital signs. Start with the T_{max} (maximum temperature over the past 24 hours) followed by the $T_{current,}$ P, BP, RR, and oxygen saturation (and weight if pertinent). Then report the intake and output information followed by a brief physical examination. The physical examination should always include the heart, lung, abdomen, and extremity examination. Don't forget about the examination of the surgical site in postoperative patients. Pay special attention to occult arrhythmias, breath sounds (to track trends in atelectasis), bowel sounds,

17

presence of abdominal distention or tympany, lower extremity edema, and peripheral pulses (use a Doppler in all vascular patients or if there is a loss of pulse that you felt before).

Example: T_{max} last night 99.5° F, $T_{current}$ is 97.8° F, pulse 66, blood pressure 115/68, respiratory rate 14. His heart has a regular rate and rhythm, and his lungs have crackles at the bases only. His abdomen is soft, nontender, and nondistended. Positive bowel sounds. No lower extremity edema. Positive dorsalis pedis and posterior tibialis pulses. The wound is clean, dry, and intact.

Step 4: Present the results of laboratory and diagnostic tests. Always check just before rounds for new laboratory or microbiology data. Old results may be mentioned if comparison is needed.

Example: The BUN this morning was 30, and the creatinine is 1.6. His white blood cell count was 10.5, and his H&H was 10.4 and 31%, and his platelet count was 105.

Step 5: The final step is the assessment and plan. Consider the status of each of the patient's problems and then state the plan. **For postoperative patients, consider postoperative recovery as one of the patient's problems or issues to be addressed here, including physical activity (increase activity level?), diet (advance diet?), and postoperative pain control (refer to the following table).**

Example: We are going to advance him from sips of clears to clear liquid diet. He said he was going to walk another two or three times today. His pain is adequately controlled. I'll touch base with oncology this morning.

Step 5 in the above list is usually the most difficult step for students. To help you with the formulation of the daily assessment and plan in postoperative patients, we have included the following table. For every postoperative patient you are following, ask yourself the questions listed. Answers to these questions will help you formulate the assessment and plan.

Issues to address in the daily management plan of postoperative patients

Questions	Comments
Does the patient's analgesic therapy need to be modified (increased or decreased)? Can the analgesic be switched to an oral formulation or even discontinued?	Adequate control of pain not only alleviates the patient's discomfort but also reduces respiratory complications and allows for early mobilization and recovery.
Can the patient's diet be advanced?	After surgery, most patients are advanced from NPO (nothing by mouth) to oral food intake based on positive responses to one or more of the following questions: Flatus reported? Bowel movements reported? Bowel sounds present? Patient hungry? Feeding is usually resumed with clear liquids and if it is well tolerated, advanced to regular diet. If there is significant delay in starting oral food intake, parenteral nutrition should be considered.

Questions	Comments
Can the patient ambulate? If already ambulating, can the activity level be increased?	Prolonged bed rest leads to muscle weakness/loss, impairment in pulmonary function, and increased risk of venous thromboembolism. For these reasons, early postoperative mobilization is encouraged.
Do intravenous fluids need to be started, modified, or stopped?	Since patients are not generally allowed to resume oral intake after surgery, intravenous fluid replacement is an important part of postoperative care.
Can any of the intravenous medications be stopped or given orally?	Medications normally given orally may have to be administered intravenously after surgery. As the patient's condition improves and oral intake is considered safe, intravenous medications can be switched to an oral formulation or discontinued if no longer necessary.
Can any tubes be removed?	The need for continued use of the nasogastric tube should be assessed daily. Indications for continued use include severe nausea/vomiting, gastric distention, prolonged ileus, and intestinal obstruction. The tube should be removed at the earliest stage possible (aspirate output < 30 mL/hour, return of bowel sounds, passing of flatus) and certainly before resuming feeding.
Can any catheters be removed?	Foley catheter can be removed when strict monitoring of urine output is no longer necessary and patient is able to urinate without assistance. Removing the catheter as early as possible is important for prevention of infection.

Questions	Comments
Can any drains be removed?	Management of drains after surgery tends to vary to some extent from one surgeon to another. Students are encouraged to consult their resident or attending physician regarding drain removal (remember to never remove a drain without asking permission!)
Can oxygen therapy be discontinued or the FIO$_2$ decreased?	
Can any sutures or staples be removed today?	Do not remove sutures or staples without permission.
Is the patient receiving prophylaxis for post-operative venous thromboembolism?	Incidence of postoperative venous thromboembolic disease can be significantly reduced if the patient receives prophylaxis. Mechanical (graduated pressure stockings, intermittent calf compression) and pharmacologic (subcutaneous unfractionated or low molecular weight heparin) techniques are available. If prophylaxis is not given to the patient for a particular reason, it should be well documented in the chart.
Does the patient need any laboratory studies today?	It has become common practice to order multiple lab tests for patients every morning. Before ordering tests, ask yourself if the test results will affect your patient's management. If the test result is unlikely to affect how you care for the patient, refrain from ordering the test.
Does the patient need any imaging tests today?	

Questions	Comments
Does the patient need physical, occupational, or respiratory therapy?	
Does the patient need social worker or discharge planner to assist with discharge and home care issues?	Consult these health care professionals early in the process to prevent or minimize delays in the patient's discharge for social reasons.

Mistake **#16**

Wasting the team's time while you take down a dressing

Many surgical patients have complicated wounds and complicated wound dressings. The dressings can often take several minutes to remove and then re-apply. Attending physicians and residents have no need to see you take down (remove) the dressing. They are interested in seeing the wound. They may or may not want to see the new dressing applied. Consistently having the dressing removed and the wound accessible for rounds will earn you extra points.

How can you accomplish this? First, gather the supplies required for dressing removal and re-application. You should either carry these supplies with you or, if allowed at your hospital, keep these in the patient's room. For wounds that are "packed" (i.e., wet-to-dry or dry-to-dry dressings that are placed on wounds left to heal by secondary intention), you will need the following:

- Suture removal kit (suture scissors and forceps)
- Kerlex or other loose-knit gauze dressing
- Large bottle (250mL to 1L) of normal saline (not sterile water)
- Plenty of 4x4 gauze dressings
- Tape (silk or paper tape)

Dressings will differ slightly among various institutions. A good rule of thumb is to have enough to form the exact same dressing as the patient currently has.

Second, you need to take down the dressing before the team arrives to see the patient. If you know the order in which patients will be seen during rounds, sneak away from your team while they are seeing the patient previous to yours. (They generally won't mind, but always check with your resident or intern prior to dressing removal.) Remove either the entire dressing or all but the last piece of dressing that is immediately over the wound. If you do this consistently, you will shine like a star on your rotation.

Mistake #17

Correcting house staff on rounds

In general, it is best to refrain from correcting residents and interns during work rounds. Doing so will clearly anger the resident or intern. Instead, speak to the resident or intern in private, immediately after rounds. An exception to this rule would be an error that could threaten the patient's safety. Outside of this, never correct the intern or resident during rounds.

Likewise, always make sure that anything you know about a patient is also known to your superior. Surgery teams operate on a hierarchy and you are expected to respect this chain of command. As the student, you should communicate new findings or results with your direct superior, which is typically an intern. It is best to do so before rounds in case the chief resident or attending physician asks the intern directly.

Mistake #18

Not knowing your patient

As far as the team is concerned, you are the patient's doctor. This means that you should be familiar with the entire hospital course and post-operative course of your patient, including the results of recent labs, imaging studies, or pathology. Check for new results before rounds. Always review imaging or pathology results with the radiologist or pathologist, respectively. Not only does this add to your learning but you will also impress your team by going one step beyond what is expected of students.

Mistake #19

Being afraid to say, "I don't know"

When a surgery resident asks you something about a patient that you don't know, the best way to reply is by saying, "I don't know but I'll find out." As an example, let's say that during rounds, your chief resident asks you for the results of a patient's complete blood count, but you don't have them. Because of your desire to look like a well-prepared student, you may be tempted to say, "I think it was normal."

You must avoid succumbing to this temptation at all costs. The best response is "I don't know, but I'll find out." This type of response demonstrates your honesty. It is better to say you don't know than to supply your resident with fabricated or incorrect information. The faulty information that you pass along can lead to certain actions or inactions, which can be harmful to the patient. Once the accuracy of your responses has been called into question, it is very difficult, if not impossible, to regain the trust of your team.

Success Tip #14
Always be honest. Do say, "I don't know" if you don't know something. Don't ever make up information.

Mistake #20

Not working with the other students as a team

Students who work well with all members of the team, including their fellow students, are more likely to impress residents and attending physicians. If another student is pimped during rounds and does not know the answer, never volunteer the answer without directly being asked. Your teammates may perceive this as showing off and be less likely to help you later. If you are asked, be modest in your answer such as "I happened to be reading…" Refrain from pimping someone higher on the ladder to flaunt your own knowledge.

Some students go to great lengths to make other students on the team look bad. Examples include prerounding and writing notes on patients other students are following (without their permission) or scrubbing in on another student's case. They are under the assumption that this type of behavior will set them apart from others, allowing them to earn a better evaluation. They are right in the sense that surgery residents and attending physicians will notice this behavior, but they are wrong in thinking it will result in a stellar evaluation. Trust on an honest and well-oiled team is the cornerstone of good surgical patient care.

Remember that residents and attending physicians have had plenty of experience working with students. If you choose to be the student who is trying to come across in a better light at the expense of your classmates, don't for a moment think that surgery residents will not pick up on it. When they do, it will certainly reflect poorly on you, and your evaluation will suffer. The frame of reference that will be used for grading is not only the three or four other students on your rotation right now, but the hundreds of other students they have worked with in the past.

Mistake **#21**

Not making a to-do list

Students often carry more patients during the surgery rotation than what they are used to. On a busy service, it can be quite difficult to remember the many things you need to do for each of your five patients, especially when they have similar problems. Regardless of how easy you think it will be to remember a particular task, write it down on your to-do list. By checking off all of the items on your list, you will be sure that nothing was forgotten. This will help you avoid the very uncomfortable situation of having to explain to the resident or attending physician why a task was never completed. As one chief surgical resident

used to say, "There are two types of surgical students—
those that write things down, and those that forget."

Mistake #22

Not paying close attention to what the residents say about your patient during work rounds

Your residents may agree with your presentation and
have nothing to add. Sometimes they may add things,
modify your plan, or change something after seeing the
patient. It's important to write these things down and pay
attention to them the next time you present. In fact, the
savvy student just writes them into the progress note that
has already been started during prerounds.

Success Tip #15

If your resident corrects you during your oral case
presentation, be sure that you understand why. Do not
repeat the error during a future presentation.

Mistake #23

Orders and notes are not signed during work rounds

By carrying the patient's chart with you during work
rounds, you can write the day's orders and have them
cosigned by the resident. If your hospital uses a
computer system, help your intern by asking which
orders he would like you to enter. This will help avoid any
delay in the implementation of the plan. Remember that,
after rounds, residents may be off to the operating room
or other places.

Mistake **#24**

Not understanding your responsibilities during afternoon rounds

During work or morning rounds, you are expected to convey patient information from the previous 24 hours to the team. For afternoon rounds, you are only expected to cover the day's events. In other words, you will focus on what has happened to the patient since morning rounds.

The order in which you present the information should be the same as the morning work rounds presentation (SOAP format). Begin by discussing the patient's symptoms and how they have changed, as well as the development of any new symptoms. This should be followed by the day's vital signs and the physical examination, which should be brief. Again, the emphasis is on how the physical examination has changed, if at all. Lab and imaging test results that were not available at the time of the work rounds presentation should be reported, as should the results of any other tests performed during the day. You will come across in a better light if you have taken the time and effort to review the test with the appropriate person (i.e., reviewing the film with radiologist or slide with the pathologist). Your presentation ends with your assessment and plan.

Your resident will also want to know whether preoperative notes have been written on patients who will have surgery the next day. Inquiries will also be made about whether postoperative checks and notes have been completed.

Success Tip #16

The start time of afternoon rounds usually varies from day to day, depending on when work in the operating room or clinic ends. If your fellow student is in the operating room with the last case of the day, help your colleague out by seeing his or her patients. Let your fellow student know how his or her patients are doing before afternoon rounds.

Success Tip #17

Morning lab test results are usually available in the late morning, well after work rounds have been completed. Be sure to inform your intern about all abnormal lab tests.

Success Tip #18

The results of pathology examinations are often not available for a few days. Check for pathology results regularly. These results often have great influence on the management and treatment of the patient's illness.

Success Tip #19

You should personally review any studies, such as x-rays and electrocardiograms.

Success Tip #20

When reporting imaging test findings, it's always better to bring the films with you for your team to review. It's even better if you can point out the abnormalities and their clinical significance in a confident manner.

Commonly Made Mistakes on the

Preoperative Note

You will be expected to write a preoperative note for every patient you are following. You are "following" a patient if you are participating in his or her care. Simply put, the purpose of the preoperative note is to convey to the readers of the chart, especially the surgical team, that the patient is ready for surgery. It answers the question "Have the things that need to be done before surgery actually been done?" In this chapter, commonly made mistakes on the preoperative note are discussed.

Mistake **#25**

Not knowing how to write a preoperative note

Most students do not know how to write a preoperative note before the start of the surgery clerkship. This is not surprising since most other rotations taken during the third year of medical school are nonsurgical. However, some of your classmates may have written preoperative notes during their obstetrics/gynecology rotation. These students will clearly be at an advantage when asked to write a preoperative note during the surgery clerkship. They may be able to write the note without any assistance or guidance whatsoever.

Students who are new to the process of preoperative note writing are often unsure how to proceed. They will ask the resident, "How do I write a preoperative note?" The resident will have to walk them through the process.

With time and experience, these students will become comfortable writing the preoperative note on their own.

Inexperienced students often don't realize that it is possible to write solid preoperative notes with very little assistance right from the start. The ability to do so would offer you some of the following advantages:

1. It would put you on par with students who already know how to write the note.

2. It would set you apart from other students who don't know how to write the note. You would be off to a better start, having impressed the resident with your initiative and preparation. Remember that surgeons are impressed with students who are independent and increase the efficiency of the team.

So how does one become comfortable with preoperative note writing if you have never done it before? Fortunately, the writing of the preoperative note is not a difficult exercise. With a little bit of preparation, a student who has never written this type of note before can do so with the polish of a seasoned veteran. The discussion in the remainder of this chapter will help you gain the knowledge needed to write the preoperative note.

Mistake **#26**

Writing the preoperative note at the wrong time

The preoperative note should be completed and in the chart *before* the patient is brought to the operating room. We recommend that you write the preoperative note the evening before an elective case. Some students choose to write or finish the note while the patient is in the preoperative holding area. We strongly discourage you from adopting this practice because more often than not, you will irk the resident or attending physician. They may ask you, "Where's the pre-op note? You know we need one to go to the OR, right?" Because your interaction with the attending physician may be limited to the OR, it's in your best interests to avoid mistakes such as this one, an error which will surely put you in a bad light with the attending physician.

Some of the advantages of writing the preoperative note the evening before surgery include the following:

- You are expected to write the preoperative note at this time. Any delay in the writing of this note will be looked upon unfavorably

- You have time to write the note at this time. Students who wait until the morning before surgery to write the note fail to recognize that mornings are often hectic. The time you thought you had for note writing may not be available to you. As an example, consider the possibility that one of your patients may take a turn for the worse, preventing you from writing the preoperative note on another patient.

- Writing the preoperative note the evening before surgery allows you to make sure that everything that needs to be done before surgery has indeed been done. It is better to realize that a necessary test, such as an EKG, was not ordered the evening before rather than the morning of the surgery. In the latter scenario, you will not have time to correct the error and surgery may have to be delayed or even cancelled.

Success Tip #21

For inpatients, write the preoperative note the evening before surgery. This will help you determine if everything that needs to be done before surgery has been done.

Mistake #27

Not having the structure or template of the preoperative note handy

Within the first few days of the rotation, you will be asked to write a preoperative note. Since you know this will happen, you should have a preoperative note template handy. By referring to the template, you should have little difficulty writing the preoperative note. You are free to copy our template and keep it with you. Or you may wish to transfer our template onto a note card, keeping it easily accessible.

Preoperative note template
Title of the note
Date and time
Preoperative diagnosis
Procedure planned
Attending surgeon
Anesthesia planned
History and physical
Allergies
Lab test data
CBC
Chem 7
PT/PTT
Urinalysis
Type & Screen or Crossmatch (#units)
EKG
Chest X-ray
Consent
NPO status/Bowel prep (if necessary)
Signature

Mistake #28

Being unclear on what to write in the preoperative note

Having the template or structure of the preoperative note is just the first step (see Mistake #27). You also need to know what to write after each element of the preoperative note (i.e., preoperative diagnosis, procedure planned, history & physical, lab test data, EKG, etc.). In the following table, we have included information that will help you create a well-written preoperative note.

Element of the preoperative note	Write...	Example
Title of note Date Time	Always start your note with the appropriate title, date, and time	"M.S. III preoperative note 2/18/04 7:30 PM"
Preoperative diagnosis	Patient's illness	"acute cholecystitis"
Procedure planned	Surgery to be performed	"laparoscopic cholecystectomy"
Attending surgeon	Name of attending surgeon	"Dr. George Roberts"
Anesthesia	Anesthesia planned	"general"
History and physical	Author of history and physical and date written	"Completed by Dr. Jones, 01/01/04."
Allergies	Medication allergy along with allergic reaction (if no medication allergies, write NKDA)	"Penicillin ('body swells up')"

Element of the preoperative note	Write...	Example
Lab test data[*]	Results of CBC, chem 7, PT/PTT, urinalysis (if performed)	Can use stick figures to convey the lab test data
Type & Screen or Crossmatch	T & S or T & C (varies with patient/surgery) along with number of units	"T & C 2 units in lab"
EKG	Results (rhythm, rate, axis, intervals, ST segment or T wave changes, other abnormalities)	"Normal sinus rhythm Normal axis No ST segment or T wave changes"
Chest X-ray[#]	Results	"Clear lung fields; normal cardiac silhouette"
Consent	Signed and in the front of the chart	"Signed by patient on 01/01/04 (in chart)"
NPO status	NPO order in chart	"NPO after midnight"
Signature	Your signature	"Alex Rodriguez, MS-3"

* When you write the preoperative note the evening before an elective case, you should include the results of the most recent lab testing (i.e., results available at the time). If the patient has another blood draw scheduled for the morning of the case, report the results in an **addendum** to the preoperative note. Do not leave blank spaces for the next morning's lab test results. Too often, these blank spaces are left empty. Furthermore, modifying a previously written note is not acceptable from a medicolegal standpoint.

Include the results of any non-standard imaging tests if they are pertinent to the patient's case (i.e., CT scan of the abdomen).

Here is an example of a preoperative note for a 25-year old woman admitted to the hospital with acute appendicitis.

01/01/04 GENERAL SURGERY "A" SERVICE PREOPERATIVE NOTE

8 PM

Preoperative diagnosis:	acute appendicitis
Procedure planned:	laparoscopic appendectomy
Attending surgeon:	Dr. Brown
Anesthesia:	general
History and physical:	written 01/01/04
Allergies:	no known drug allergies (NKDA)
CBC:	(1/01/04): *insert stick figure here*
Chemistry:	(1/01/04): *insert stick figure here*
Urinalysis:	(1/01/04): no WBCs, nitrite negative, no blood
Type and screen:	completed 01/01/04
EKG:	1/01/04): not indicated
CXR:	(1/01/04): no evidence of acute cardiopulmonary disease
Consent:	signed by patient on 01/01/04, witnessed and in chart
	NPO as of midnight

Joe Lister
MS-3

Mistake **#29**

Not realizing that something important is missing prior to surgery

As stated in the introduction to this chapter, the preoperative note answers the question "Have the things that need to be done before surgery actually been done?" As you are gathering the information and writing the preoperative note, you may find that some information is missing. For example, some laboratory testing may not have been performed. At times, the testing may not have been performed because indications to do so were lacking in that particular patient. Sometimes, though, the test(s) are indicated but because of one error or another, they were not performed. In these latter cases, if you are able to pick up on these errors, you can order the necessary tests, thereby preventing a delay or cancellation of the procedure because of an incomplete preoperative evaluation. In the following table, we describe the indications for preoperative testing. If you feel that a test has not been obtained because of error, be sure to let your resident know.

Does my patient need preoperative measurement of ...	Yes, if ...
Hemoglobin	● Significant blood loss is anticipated during surgery ● Clinical manifestations of anemia are present

Does my patient need preoperative measurement of ...	Yes, if ...
Electrolytes	● Condition(s) associated with electrolyte abnormalities are present (Examples include diarrhea, diabetes mellitus, renal disease, diuretic use, steroid use, adrenal disease, those unable to provide history, SIADH, diabetes insipidus, and severe liver disease.)
Renal function tests	● Diabetes mellitus or renal disease is present ● Patient is undergoing major surgery ● Patient will be receiving nephrotoxic medications ● Hypotension is likely or anticipated ● Age > 50 years (widespread consensus lacking on this indication)
Glucose	● Diabetes mellitus or adrenal disease is present ● Patient is on corticosteroid therapy
Liver function tests	● History of liver disease or hepatitis
PT/PTT	● History is compatible with bleeding disorder (or known bleeding disorder) ● Patient has condition associated with bleeding (liver disease) ● Patient has been receiving an oral anticoagulant ● Patient is unable to provide history
Urinalysis	● Urinary tract instrumentation is likely
TSH	● Patient has or is suspected of having thyroid disease

Does my patient need preoperative measurement of …	Yes, if …
Chest x-ray	• Signs and/or symptoms of cardiopulmonary disease are present • Age > 60 years No need to perform study if one has been done in the past six months (unless there has been a change in the patient's status).
EKG	• Patient has known cardiac disease • Patient is suspected of having cardiac disease • Men > 45 years of age • Women > 55 years of age • Patient has systemic disease associated with cardiac disease/complications (e.g., hypertension, diabetes mellitus) • Risk factors for electrolyte abnormalities are present (e.g., diuretic use) • Patient is undergoing major surgery No need to perform EKG if one has been done in the past month (unless there has been a change in the patient's status).

Mistake #30

Not helping your intern write other patients' preoperative notes

Surgical interns and residents are extremely busy. With so many patients on the service, they are often pulled in many different directions. As a student, you can help lighten their load in a variety of ways. Writing preoperative notes on patients you are not following is one way to do so. If you are aware of the next day's OR schedule, take the initiative and write the preoperative notes for the intern. If you are not sure of the schedule, ask the intern and then volunteer to write the notes. These types of actions show the team that you are indeed a team player.

When writing preoperative notes for others, do not take it to an extreme. What do we mean by this? We urge you not to write preoperative notes for patients assigned to other students unless they ask for your assistance or you have their permission. It's never acceptable to show up other students.

Mistake **#31**

Not receiving feedback on the quality of your preoperative notes

In a perfect world, the surgical resident would review the preoperative note with you. We can tell you that this often does not happen. Quite often, preoperative notes written by students are simply cosigned and mistakes are corrected without any feedback being given regarding the quality of the notes. Do not be afraid to seek feedback if you find yourself in this type of situation.

If you have not been given feedback, first start by looking over your preoperative note to see if the resident has added or changed anything. If so, try to understand why the information was added or changed because this understanding will clearly be of benefit to you when writing future notes. Then, discuss your note with the resident (at an appropriate time), asking him or her specific questions. Instead of "What did you think about my preoperative note?" consider asking the following types of questions:

- How can I improve the quality of my preoperative notes?

- Were there any major omissions?

- I noticed that you added ... to my note. Do you recommend that I include this information in future notes or was this addition something that pertains only to this patient?

- I noticed that you changed _____ in my note. I'm not sure that I understand why. Can you fill me in?

Since the preoperative note is just one type of note you will be writing during the surgical clerkship, you will want to solicit feedback regarding the quality of your other notes, including operative, postoperative, and daily progress notes. You may use the same questions listed above to identify areas that require improvement.

Commonly Made Mistakes on the

Brief Operative Note

You will be expected to write a brief operative note for every patient you are following. You are "following" a patient if you are participating in his or her care. At the end of an operation, the brief operative note should be written in the progress notes section of the chart. The main purpose of the note is to inform chart readers of the events that occurred in the OR.

The resident or attending physician will also dictate a full operative note. Although the dictated note contains the same information found in the brief operative note, the former is much more detailed than the latter. Since it usually takes several days for the dictated report to be transcribed and placed in the chart, readers of the chart will rely on your brief operative note to learn particulars about the surgery. For example, if your patient develops acute renal failure one day after surgery, the nephrology service (if consulted) will be very interested in the patient's input and output (during surgery) you have reported in the operative note. In this chapter, we will discuss mistakes made on the operative note.

Mistake **#32**

Not knowing how to write a brief operative note

Unless you have rotated through obstetrics/gynecology prior to your surgery clerkship, you probably don't know how to write an operative note. Most students learn to write the operative note at the end of the first operation they participate in. What typically happens is that the resident will turn to the student and ask him or her to write the operative note. The student, having never written one, will say, "Can you show me how to write one?"

Instead of being the student described above, with a little bit of preparation, you can easily write an operative note when your resident asks you to do so for the first time. Your resident will be impressed if you are able to write an operative note with little instruction at this point in your rotation.

Mistake **#33**

Not having the template of the operative note handy

With time and experience, you may not need to refer to a template for operative note writing. Having a template is particularly useful, however, for students who have never written an operative note or are in the early part of their clerkship. On the next page, we have included our operative note template. You may wish to copy the template and keep it somewhere readily accessible. Some students prefer to write the skeleton of the operative note in the patient's progress notes before the surgery. After surgery, these students simply fill in the blanks.

Operative note template

Title of note
Date/time
Pre-op diagnosis
Post-op diagnosis
Procedure and indication
Surgeon (attending)
First assistant (most senior resident)
Second assistant
Student
Anesthesia
Input (IV fluids + blood products)
Output (EBL + UO + drains + any
    other)
Drains
Findings
Specimen/cultures
Complications
Disposition

EBL = estimated blood loss
UO = urine output

Mistake #34

Not knowing what to write in the operative note

Having the template of the operative note is just the first step (see Mistake #33). You also need to know what to write after each element of the operative note (i.e., preoperative diagnosis, postoperative diagnosis, procedure, EBL, input, etc.). In the following tables, we have included information that will help you create a well-written operative note.

In the following table, we provide an example of a completed operative note. Please keep in mind that there may be some variation in the writing of this note from one institution to another. It is best to talk with the resident to determine what is preferred.

01/01/04 GENERAL SURGERY "A" SERVICE: BRIEF OPERATIVE NOTE

3 PM

Pre-operative diagnosis: colon cancer

Post-operative diagnosis: colon cancer

Procedure: left hemicolectomy with en-bloc partial bladder resection

Attending surgeon: Dr. Brown

First assistant: Dr. Jones

Student: Harry Cushing MS-3

Anesthesia: Dr. N. Tubate. General anesthesia endotracheal tube

Input: 3L normal saline + 250 mL albumin + 2U pRBCs.

Output: 550 mL EBL + 800 mL UO + 150 mL NG tube.

Findings: firm mass in left colon with gross invasion of the dome of the bladder; no liver or peritoneal metastases appreciated.

Specimens: left colon and bladder sent to pathology for permanent section and staging.

Drains: Foley draining to gravity; nasogastric tube to low intermittent wall suction (LIWS); Jackson-Pratt drain in left paracolic gutter to bulb suction.

Complications: no known complications.

Disposition: to post-anesthesia care unit (PACU) in stable condition, extubated

Harry Cushing
MS-3

Mistake **#35**

Not knowing how to describe operative findings

Students are often unsure of what to write under "findings." Start by focusing on the reason the operation was performed. For example, was the appendix inflamed? Perforated? Was any gross tumor invasion seen? Any anatomical anomalies noted? You may include both unexpected findings and expected findings. You should consider what to write and then run this by the resident to make sure it is accurate. This approach is better than simply turning to the resident and saying "I'm not sure what I should write here."

Mistake **#36**

Not knowing what to write under "complications"

Write "no known complications" when no problems occurred during the case. If there were problems, it is best to talk with the resident and/or attending surgeon before writing anything. Do not write anything other than "no known complications" without talking to the rest of the surgery team.

Mistake **#37**

Not writing the postoperative orders

After surgery, postoperative orders need to be written. At some institutions, students are expected to write these orders. At other places, no such expectations exist and order writing is the responsibility of the attending physician or resident. Even if you are not expected to write postoperative orders, we encourage you to do so. Your superiors will certainly be impressed with your initiative. After you have written the orders, you will have the opportunity to discuss them with your resident or attending physician. The ensuing discussion will help you gain a better understanding of the patient's illness and important aspects of postoperative care. Remember also that there will come a time when you are responsible for order writing and the experiences you have as a student will undoubtedly help you when you become an intern.

Mistake #38

Not having a mnemonic for postoperative order writing

Nurses and other healthcare professionals rely on the postoperative orders to provide appropriate patient care during the postoperative period. What is ordered will vary from patient to patient depending on the patient's condition, surgery, and other medical problems. However, the components of each patient's postoperative orders are the same. A useful way to remember these components is to use the mnemonic ABC VANDALISM, the same mnemonic used for admission order writing. By using this or a similar mnemonic, the student can be confident that all the components or elements of the postoperative orders will be included.

Mnemonic for postoperative orders
Date and time
Admit to
Because (diagnosis)
Condition
Vital signs
Activity
Nursing
Diet
Allergies
Laboratory tests
IV orders
Special orders
Medications
Signature/name

Mistake #39

Not knowing how to write the postoperative orders

Having the mnemonic handy for postoperative order writing is just the first step in the process. You also need to know what to write after each component of the postoperative orders. The table below provides guidance with postoperative order writing.

Don't lose sight of the fact that, at this point in your career you are not expected to be proficient with the writing of the postoperative orders. What is more important is that you take the initiative to write the orders, have a mnemonic ready, and have some understanding of what to write after each component of the orders. With that being said, don't be surprised if your resident or attending physician adds, modifies, deletes, or changes your orders.

Do, however, learn from the changes that are made.

Component of postoperative orders	What to write
Date/time	Orders should always begin with the date and time
Admit to	Location patient is being transported to. In most cases, this will be the recovery room (PACU). Often, the service and the attending physician the patient is admitted or assigned to are included.
Condition	Condition of the patient (e.g., fair, critical)
Vital signs	Specify frequency of vital signs measurement. Often, vital sign parameters are written to inform the nurse when the physician should be notified of abnormalities of the blood pressure, respiratory rate, pulse, and temperature.
Activity	Generally, patients will be at bed rest immediately after surgery and activity status will then differ depending on the procedure

Component of postoperative orders	What to write
Nursing	Indicate what nursing staff has to do for the patient. Include the following information (if pertinent):
	I & O (when it should be recorded)
	Drains/catheters
	Name all tubes, drains, and catheters
	Indicate frequency of output measurement
	Indicate how they should be maintained, cared, and positioned
	Indicate type of suction (to low wall suction [LWS], to gravity, to bulb)
	Incentive spirometry
	Bedside blood sugar measurement
	Encouragement of deep breathing and coughing
	Supplemental oxygen
	Wound care instructions
Diet	Generally, patients are NPO after abdominal surgery
Allergies	Record any medication allergies (along with the reaction)

Component of postoperative orders	What to write
Laboratory tests	List lab tests to be ordered as well as when they should be obtained. Routine lab test orders are discouraged. Obtain only those tests whose results may affect patient management.
IV orders	Generally, postoperative patients are initially given LR/normal saline at maintenance, depending on their intraoperative resuscitation, and changed to 1/2 normal saline thereafter
Special orders	Include orders that do not fit neatly under other components.
Medications	For every medication, indicate: Name (generic name preferred) Dosage Route Frequency or time of administration For PRN medications, specify the indication. In addition to the patient's baseline medications, don't forget to include antibiotics and medications for pain, nausea, fever, and DVT/peptic ulcer disease prophylaxis. Consider writing an insulin sliding scale for diabetic patients.
Name/signature	Sign the orders and print your name underneath the signature.

In the following table, we provide an example of postoperative orders.

01/01/04 5 p.m.	General Surgery "A" Service: Postoperative Orders
Admit to	Surgery Ward, Dr. J. Murray's service (Transplant Surgery)
Diagnosis	S/P laparascopic nephrectomy for living related kidney donation
Condition	Fair
Allergies	NKDA
Vital Signs	Please record BP, P, RR, and T q8 hours
Activity	Activity as tolerated. Head of bed to 30 degrees when in bed. Out of bed in AM

Nursing	Please record I/Os q8 hours
	Foley to gravity
	Nasogastric tube to low intermittent suction
	Notify Transplant Service house officer if:
	  -T > 100.5 F
	  -P > 100 or < 60
	  -SBP > 150 or < 100
	  -DBP > 100 or < 60
	  -RR > 25 or < 15
	  -Urine output < 30 mL/hour
	TED hose and SCDs to both legs at all times while in bed
	Incentive spirometry q1 hour while awake
	Encourage deep breathing and coughing
	Please do not remove dressings

Diet	Sips of clears
IV orders	Heplock

Medications	Darvon 65 mg po q4 hours PRN pain
	Tylenol 650 mg po q8 hours PRN fever > 100.5 F
	Bisacodyl 10 mg po qd
	Enoxaprin 40 mg SQ qd
	Ceftriaxone 1 mg IV qd X one dose
	Ranitidine 50 mg IV q8 hours
Laboratory tests	Serum biochemistry and CBC with platelets upon admission to the unit and q AM
Special orders	Chest x-ray upon arrival to PACU (reason: s/p left subclavian central line placement)
Name/ Signature	Harry Cushing MS-3

Mistake #40

Not paying close attention as the end of the case nears

As the end of a surgery case nears, the attending physician may pass along some important information to the resident. The attending may comment on some aspects of the patient's postoperative care. For example, a certain antibiotic or analgesic may be preferred. Some attending physicians may be very specific with their requests. You should pay close attention to these comments because you will certainly want your postoperative orders to include these requests. Your initiative and attention to detail will certainly impress your resident and attending physician.

Postoperative Note

A wide variety of problems can develop in the postoperative patient, many of which are quite serious. It is important to detect these problems, which is why a member of the team must evaluate the patient postoperatively. The findings of the postoperative evaluation should be included in the postoperative note. In this chapter, we will discuss mistakes made on the postoperative note.

Mistake #41

Not writing the postoperative note

You should write the postoperative note for every patient that you are following. Stellar surgery students often evaluate the patient on their own and write a postoperative note. They then give their resident a brief verbal summary of the patient's condition before seeing the patient together.

The postoperative note is typically written the evening after surgery. It should not be written any earlier than four hours after the operation; the patient should be seen before that in the PACU.

Mistake **#42**

Not having a template for the postoperative note

With experience, you will become familiar with the elements of the postoperative note, so that you may not need to refer to a template. Early on in the rotation, it is helpful to carry a card with the postoperative note template on it (or you can choose to copy our template below) to refer to when writing the postoperative note.

Postoperative note template

Title of the note
Date and time of the note
Procedure
Subjective
Level of consciousness/mental
  status
Pain control
Vital signs
  Temperature
  Heart rate
  Blood pressure
  Respiratory rate
Urine output
Drain output
Physical examination (including
  inspection of wound/drain)
Laboratory/radiographic data
Assessment/plan

Mistake **#43**

Not knowing what to write in the postoperative note

Having the template or structure of the postoperative note is just the first step (see mistake #42). You also need to know what to write after each element of the postoperative note. In the following table, we have included information that will help you create a well-written postoperative note.

Element of the post-operative note	Write ...	Example
Title of note Date Time	Always start your note with the appropriate title, date, and time	"M.S. III postoperative note 2/19/04 10:24 PM"
Procedure	Name of procedure and indication	"s/p cadaveric kidney transplant"
Level of consciousness/ mental status	Indicate if the patient is alert, oriented, lethargic, somnolent, or unresponsive	"Alert and oriented."
Pain control	Adequate, poor, etc. Consider describing means of analgesia.	"Pain is well tolerated with morphine PCA."
Vital signs	List T, HR, RR, BP.	"T_c=37.5C, P=70, RR=20, BP=135/ 70."

Element of the post-operative note	Write ...	Example
Urine output	List urine output since surgery (> 30 mL/hour or 0.5 cc/kg body weight/hour is adequate for most adult patients depending on the surgery).	"UO=200 cc clear yellow urine."
Drain output	List location and type of drain as well as quantity and quality of fluid.	"Jackson-Pratt drain in R pelvis has drained 10 mLs of serosanguinous fluid."
Physical exam	Brief physical exam (i.e. cardiac, pulmonary, abdominal, neurological exam; examine area of surgery).	"Heart RRR. Lungs clear, good inspiratory effort. Abdomen minimally tender, non-distended. R pelvic wound dressed; minimal blood staining on dressing."
Laboratory/ radiographic data	Write down results of any postoperative labs or imaging tests.	See example below.
Assessment/plan	Brief outline of overnight plan (i.e. next 12-24 hours).	See example below.

In the following table, we have provided an example of a postoperative note written by a third-year surgery student.

General Surgery "A" Service: Postoperative Note	
01/01/04 10 p.m.	52 year-old man s/p left hemicolectomy and partial bladder resection for locally-advanced colon cancer. Reports adequate pain control with patient-controlled anesthesia (PCA). Has not yet ambulated. Denies nausea or vomiting.
Objective:	
General	awake, alert and oriented. Appears comfortable.
Vitals	T_{max} = 37.5°C, Tc = 37.6°C, RR = 14, P = 66, P = 130/80
Output	200 cc UO (~0.7cc/kg/hour for 4 hrs); 50 cc per NG tube.
Heart	regular rate and rhythm
Lungs	clear to auscultation; good inspiratory effort
Abdomen	non-distended. Absent bowel sounds.
Wound	dressing in place; minimal blood staining.
Extremities	TED hose and sequential compression devices (SCDs) in place on both lower extremities
Postoperative labs/imaging:	Glucose 156
Assessment/ Plan:	52 year-old man s/p left hemicolectomy for locally advanced colon cancer. Will continue PCA for pain control. Patient encouraged to use incentive spirometry. Continue intravenous fluids and keep NPO. Out-of-bed in morning. Medical oncology service consulted; will see patient in morning regarding adjuvant therapy. H&H, serum biochemistries pending for AM.
Alex Carrel MS-3	

Mistake **#44**

Not looking at the wound dressing at the post-operative check

One of the main reasons for a post-operative check is to assess the surgical site within a few hours of the operation. Wounds and closures will vary from clean incisions, to traumatic wounds, to those being left open to heal by secondary intention. Being able to assess the wound takes experience and the more wounds you see, the more you get a feeling for what is normal vs. abnormal (e.g. wound erythema vs. cellulitis). Therefore, assess every wound and describe exactly what you see to get an arsenal of experience.

The key question you are trying to answer is "Are there any signs of hemorrhage?" These signs may include a blood-soaked dressing, a tender and distended abdomen, or a large hematoma. The house staff will probably not want you to remove the dressing, but you should look at the dressing itself and palpate the area immediately surrounding the wound (fluctuance would suggest the presence of a fluid collection or hematoma). If you notice signs suggestive of wound hemorrhage or hematoma in the immediate postoperative period, notify your intern. Assessment of the patient's wound, including the site and severity of the bleeding, will allow the team to make decisions regarding the need for re-exploration, surgical evacuation, or pressure dressings.

Mistake **#45**

Not paying attention to postoperative level of consciousness in an extubated patient

When extubated, postoperative patients should be arousable and coherent. A diminished level of consciousness may be a significant problem. While it is not unusual for the patient to be sleepy, he or she should be easily aroused to voice or touch. At a minimum, the patient should be able to respond to simple questions (i.e. yes-no questions) or follow simple directions. Don't just attribute a diminished level of consciousness to the lingering effect of general anesthesia – let the house staff know if you have any doubts at all.

Mistake **#46**

Answering questions that should be left to the resident or attending surgeon

Patients often do not remember discussions they may have had with the surgery team in the recovery room or PACU following surgery. As the effects of the anesthesia wear off, quite naturally, they will be interested in knowing what happened during surgery. To them, it may seem that your arrival for the postoperative check-up is the first time they have seen a member of the surgical team after surgery. In reality, they have probably been tended to by various members of the team but do not recall these interactions or the discussions that have already taken place about their surgery.

Therefore, it is not surprising for patients to want to discuss the procedure with you. You should be careful, however, when answering these questions. Quite often, answers to these questions are better left to the surgery resident or attending surgeon. In many cases, you may not have a full understanding of the patient's condition, in which case your responses may be off the mark. In other cases, a delicate approach by someone who has the best rapport and longest relationship with the patient may be necessary (like the attending surgeon). It is not your job as a student to deliver important or potentially devastating information to the patient.

Mistake #47

Failing to check the lab test/EKG results (if they are done) as soon as they are back in the PACU

The Post Anesthesia Care Unit, also known as PACU or recovery room, is the area of the hospital where patients are transported to after surgery. Here, patients begin the process of recovering from the immediate effects of anesthesia. From the PACU, patients are either discharged home or to the hospital floor.

While in the PACU, patients may develop a variety of problems. Common PACU problems are listed in the following box.

Common PACU problems

Delayed awakening
Postoperative pain
Postoperative delirium
Postoperative agitation
Postoperative nausea/vomiting
Pulmonary problems
    Hypoventilation
    Hypoxemia
    Airway obstruction
    Stridor/wheezing
    Aspiration
    Pulmonary edema
Cardiovascular problems
    Hypotension
    Hypertension
    Myocardial ischemia/infarction
    Arrhythmia
Renal problems
    Oliguria
    Hematuria
    Urinary retention
    Polyuria
    Electrolyte/metabolic abnormalities
Hypothermia
Hyperthermia
Prolonged neuromuscular weakness
Blood transfusion reactions
Ventilator management

Frequent checking for the return of any postoperative lab tests is an important part of postoperative patient care. The physiologic response to surgery and intraoperative fluid management cause fluid shifts between the extracellular and intracellular milieu, which may result in the development of electrolyte disturbances. These often need to be corrected in the PACU. Failure to do so can result in severe metabolic imbalance with potentially catastrophic results. Furthermore, postoperative hematocrit/hemoglobin, coagulation studies, and other labs (if ordered) need to be checked immediately since abnormalities may be clues to possible complications. Their recognition will aid in the postoperative management of these patients. Be sure to let your resident know of any abnormal findings.

It is common for perioperative myocardial infarction to present asymptomatically. In the immediate postoperative period, the EKG is often the best tool to assess for cardiac ischemia/infarction. The EKG should be done expeditiously in selected patient populations and interpreted as soon as it comes off the machine. This will allow for an early diagnosis of active ischemia or infarction, thereby preventing an all-too-common occurrence—that is, the failure to quickly diagnose and manage active ischemia or infarction because no one looked at the EKG in a timely manner.

As a student, you must understand that your care of the postoperative patient is not interrupted by the patient's brief stay in the PACU. In other words, you do not resume care when the patient is transferred out of the PACU but the patient is very much yours during their stay in the PACU. Your vigilance and attention to detail may uncover some of the problems discussed above.

Commonly Made Mistakes on the

Daily Progress Note

You will be expected to write a daily progress note for every patient you are following. You are "following" a patient if you are participating in his or her care. The purpose of the daily progress note is to update readers of the patient's hospital course since the last progress note was written. Other health care professionals rely heavily on the daily progress note, especially the assessment and plan, to learn not only about the patient's progress but also about the current diagnostic and therapeutic plan. In this chapter, mistakes students commonly make on the daily progress note are discussed.

Mistake **#48**

Using an improper format

Daily progress notes should be written using the **SOAP** format. SOAP is an acronym for "**S**ubjective, **O**bjective, **A**ssessment, and **P**lan." In the subjective portion of the note, the patient's complaints are listed. In the objective section, the physical examination and laboratory data are reported. The note concludes with your assessment and plan. Notes that do not follow this order are considered disorganized and difficult to follow. The next box provides a step by step approach to daily progress note writing. By following the steps, you will be able to produce a well-written daily progress note.

Step-by-step approach to the writing of the daily progress note

Step 1: Start by writing the heading. The heading should include the date/time, title of the note, the surgery service you are a member of, and your rank. The hospital day # should follow. For the postoperative patient, include the postoperative day # (POD) as well. If the patient is taking an antibiotic, many surgeons prefer the name and the number of days of antibiotic therapy to be listed after the POD #.

Example: 2/3/04 6 AM Surgery Service A MS3 Progress Note Hospital Day #2, POD #2 s/p appendectomy

Step 2: Write the subjective information. Include new complaints/symptoms as well as any change in old complaints/symptoms. In the postoperative patient, don't forget to write about pain (location, severity, duration, quality, effectiveness of analgesic therapy), ambulation/activity, bowel habits (presence/absence, constipation/diarrhea, flatus, bowel movements), appetite, diet (tolerating?), and incentive spirometry use.

Example: Patient does report some peri-incisional pain but states that his pain is fairly well controlled with PCA. No flatus or bowel movements. He is ambulating without difficulty. He has been using the incentive spirometer every few hours.

Step 3: Write down the vital signs (usually recorded on the bedside chart). Include the T_{max} (maximum temperature over the past 24 hours and when it occurred), $T_{current}$, pulse, respiratory rate, and blood pressure. For the latter 3 vital signs, also include ranges if there has been significant fluctuation. Oxygen saturation (as well as the amount of supplemental oxygen being administered) and weight should be reported, if pertinent to the patient.

Example: T_{max} - 99.7°F $T_{current}$ - 99.2°F P - 66 RR - 14
BP - 115/68

Step 4: Write down the I/Os (Ins & Outs) over the past 24 hours (I/Os are usually recorded on the bedside chart). The total input includes oral and intravenous fluids. The total output may include urine, stool, emesis, drain, and NG tube output. Each drain output should be recorded separately as well (don't forget to specify hours and the character of the fluid that is draining).

Example: 24 hour I/O 2300/2200, Urine output 1400

Step 5: Report brief physical examination. Comment on general appearance as well as heart, lung, abdominal, and extremity exams. Focus also on the area of interest (why patient was hospitalized). In the postoperative patient, comment on the condition of the incision site/wound (appearance, discharge, tenderness).

Example: General - Awake, alert, and cooperative
Heart - RRR, nl S1 and S2, no murmurs/rubs/gallops
Lungs - CTA bilaterally
Abd - NABS, NT, ND
Ext - No clubbing/cyanosis/edema, SCDs in place
Incision site - Clean/dry/intact

Step 6: List laboratory test results (use stick figures, if possible) that were done over the past 24 hours, which were not documented in a prior note. You may include previously reported lab test results if trends are important. Don't forget to include the date and time of all lab test results. If results are not available, write "pending" (can be charted later as an addendum).

Example: Hemoglobin 10.4 (yesterday 10.9)
BUN 13
Creatinine 1.1

Step 7: List the results of any other diagnostic studies (i.e., radiology, cardiology, pathology). Include the date and time of the study. Offer your own interpretation for EKG/imaging tests if the official report is pending (also write "official report pending").

Step 8: Write the assessment and plan. Start with a short statement of the patient's age, gender, and reason for being in the hospital. For both the preoperative and postoperative patient, discuss the patient's general condition (significant improvement? new concerns?). Then discuss the diagnostic and therapeutic plan.

For the postoperative patient, the plan for the day should also include issues related to pain control (increase/decrease/discontinue/switch from PCA to po?), diet (advance?), patient activity (increase activity level?), incentive spirometry, antibiotics (discontinue?), drains (discontinue?), staples (discontinue?), intravenous fluids (change or discontinue?), and lines/catheters (discontinue?).

Example: *Patient is a 72-year-old man who is POD #2 s/p appendectomy for acute appendicitis*
- *Overall doing well*
- *Encourage continued ambulation*
- *Encourage continued use of incentive spirometry*
- *Will switch from PCA to po analgesia*
- *Continue NPO*
- *Continue DVT prophylaxis with SCDs*

Mistake **#49**

Note is too long

Daily progress notes written by surgery residents are brief, sometimes just several lines in length. Notes written by students should clearly be longer. How long should they be? While we cannot give you a length that would be appropriate for every patient, lengthy notes are discouraged. This tends to be a problem for students who have rotated through the Internal Medicine clerkship where writing daily progress notes of two or three pages is not unusual. Ask your resident or intern if you are not sure how long your notes should be.

Success Tip #22
In general, daily progress notes should not exceed one page in length.

Mistake **#50**

Not finishing the note in the morning

In contrast to other clerkships, the daily progress note should be completed before or at the end of work rounds. The savvy student simply writes the daily progress note during prerounds when he or she is gathering information about the patient. The information gathered essentially forms the basis of the daily progress note. During morning work rounds with the rest of the surgery team, additional information can be added to the progress note if necessary. For example, during work rounds, the surgery residents may take the following actions:

- Uncover a complaint that was not reported to you during prerounds
- Make note of a physical examination finding that you did not appreciate
- Decide to order a lab test or diagnostic study you had not considered
- Change or add to your plan

You can simply add this information to the note that you have already started.

Success Tip #23

Leave some room at the end of the note for the intern or attending physician. They will often have something to add.

Mistake #51

Incorrectly numbering the postoperative day

This is clearly one of the most common mistakes students make when writing the daily progress note. Remember that the day of the operation is postoperative day # 0 (POD # 0). The day *after* the operation is postoperative day # 1.

Mistake #52

Not including the patient's medication list

Surgery daily progress notes should include the patient's medication list, including any analgesic or antibiotic medications. For antibiotics, it is important to include the number of days the patient has been taking the medication. The medication list should be placed either at the top or the side of the progress note.

Mistake #53

Writing an incorrect plan

The assessment and plan is usually the most difficult part of note writing for students. Your first step is to have a clear understanding of what the assessment and plan is. During morning work rounds, many different plans or options may have been considered. Before writing the plan, you need to know which plan is to be implemented. If you are not sure, do not hesitate to ask the intern or resident. Sometimes students are knowledgeable about the day's plan but are not able to explain the rationale behind it. If you find yourself in this position, spend some time with the intern or resident to gain a better understanding.

When writing the plan, avoid writing phrases or words like "will consider" or "possible." Instead, your wording should reflect your commitment to a plan. For complicated patients, your resident may prefer the plan be written in a systems based format. In this format, each problem is a system. An example:

Pulmonary

Gastrointestinal

Cardiovascular

Wile some prefer to list the systems in a particular order irrespective of the patient's primary problem, others list the systems in descending order of importance.

Next to each system, relevant issues are discussed. For example, if the patient is hospitalized with acute cholecystitis, the assessment and plan may be listed as follows:

Gastrointestinal: Acute cholecystitis - symptoms and signs improved. Continue NPO, intravenous antibiotics, and intravenous fluids.

Success Tip #24
Never discuss the plan with the patient until it has been approved by the team.

Success Tip #25
If you are uncertain of the plan, hold off on completing this portion of your note until you discuss it with the team.

Success Tip #26
Be sure to have your intern sign your note during or immediately after work rounds.

Mistake #54

Not adding information as an addendum

Additional information about the patient (lab test results, diagnostic study results, consultant recommendations) may become available later in the day. The writing of the progress note should not be delayed until these results return. This additional information can be charted, if necessary, as an addendum.

The addendum should be written in the next available space in the progress notes section of the chart. The addendum should begin with a title, "Addendum to the progress note of (date)" followed by the additional information. Avoid writing an addendum in the margin because it is messy. It may also look suspicious should the chart be reviewed for any medicolegal reasons.

Mistake #55

Scribbling out errors

Errors in the daily progress note should not be scribbled or blocked out. The appropriate way of handling an error is to cross it out with a single horizontal line. The word "error" should be written next to it along with the date and your initials.

Mistake #56

Making premature diagnoses

Do not make premature diagnoses in the chart. Describe a large descending colon mass as a "mass," not a cancer, until there is tissue diagnosis confirming it to be cancer. Alternatively, you can write "left colon mass rule out cancer."

Before asking the intern or resident to review/cosign your daily progress note, ask yourself the following questions:

1. Have I written down the date and time of the note?
2. Have I titled the note?
3. Have I included the subjective data?
4. Have I included the vital signs?
5. Have I included the patient's total intake?
6. Have I included the patient's total output?
7. Have I listed each component of the intake (e.g., intravenous, po, etc.) and output (e.g., urine, drain, etc.) individually?
8. Have I addressed the important aspects of the physical examination (heart, lung, abdomen, extremity, area of interest)
9. Have I described the wound?
10. Are all laboratory test results listed?
11. Are the results of all other diagnostic studies noted?
12. Is there an assessment before every plan?
13. Is the plan specific?
14. Have I organized the information in the appropriate manner?
15. Have I signed the note?

Mistake **#57**

Not writing the procedure note

A procedure note needs to be written after all procedures (successful or not). Examples of procedures that require notes include central line placement, chest tube placement, paracentesis, thoracentesis, arthrocentesis, arterial line placement, and lumbar puncture. If you are involved in the procedure or even if you are simply observing, volunteer to write the procedure note. It shows initiative on your part. The content of the procedure note is described in the following box.

Content of the procedure note
Procedure performed Indications Summary of informed consent discussion (i.e., risks) Description of procedure Results of procedure Complications

Commonly Made Mistakes in the

Operating Room

After completing work rounds, the day continues in the operating room. As a medical student, you should participate in the operating room as much as you can. This is your opportunity to take part in surgery and although your role may seem limited, it is certainly important. Participating in the surgery of patients you are following is a valuable part of the learning process during the clerkship. Even with patients you are not following, being present in the operating room will help solidify information you have read about the patient's surgical condition.

Because other rotations, except for obstetrics/ gynecology, do not have an operating room component, the experience, at first, may seem very overwhelming. Students are often unsure of how to dress, scrub, gown, glove, prepare the patient for surgery, and maintain the sterile field. Unfamiliarity with the operating room setting creates an environment in which mistakes can be easily made. Even as a student's comfort level increases, mistakes continue to be made in other areas, such as attending interactions. In this chapter, we will discuss the mistakes students make in the operating room.

Mistake **#58**

Not attending the operating room orientation

Almost all surgery clerkships will have an operating room orientation, usually on the first day of the rotation.

Attendance is usually mandatory but even if it is not stated as such, it behooves you to be present. During the orientation, you will learn about the principles of aseptic technique and the correct way to scrub, gown, and glove before surgery. This is the first step towards becoming more comfortable in the operating room.

Mistake #59

Not paying close attention to what is said and done during the operating room orientation

We have seen many students lose focus during the operating room orientation. Although it is easy to drift off, you must pay close attention to what is being said. Unless you have already rotated through the gynecology clerkship, it's unlikely that you have had significant exposure to the operating room. It is precisely this unfamiliarity that leads to many operating room errors. These mistakes have the potential to cause great harm to the patient and, in some cases, they can be a significant hazard to you as well as the rest of the surgical team.

During orientation, you will learn about the rules of the operating room. These rules are in place to ensure that everyone adheres to the principles of aseptic technique. Surgery disrupts the skin, which is the body's barrier against infection and disease. With the body's defenses lowered, microorganisms now have access to the inner tissues with the chance to proliferate and cause infection. To prevent infection from developing during surgery, it is necessary to follow the rules of aseptic technique. By becoming familiar with these rules, you will be less likely to make mistakes that might subject the patient to infection.

Mistake #60

Not being in the operating room every day

There should not be a day that you are not in the operating room. Exceptions to this rule would be days during which there are no cases scheduled or when your help is required on the floors or in the clinics.

You will notice that your surgical residents look forward to being in the operating room. They will appreciate it if you show the same enthusiasm when you are presented with the opportunity to participate in a patient's surgery. If you are ever asked to participate in a case, your answer should always be a resounding and enthusiastic "Yes!"

Being an active participant in the operating room also allows you to interact more closely with surgical attendings. Although you will likely have contact with attending physicians on the floors, in the clinics, and during conferences, demands on their time may limit your interactions in these settings. In the operating room, attending physicians are shielded from their other responsibilities, allowing them to engage in a discussion about the patient's case with you.

Mistake #61

Finishing the rotation without seeing the core important cases

Being in the operating room is a rare opportunity to correlate symptoms and signs with direct visualization of pathology and corresponding anatomy. Your involvement in cases from diagnosis to the operating room will help train your clinical eye, acquiring skills that will benefit you regardless of the field of medicine you pursue as a career. There are some cases that are considered essential to the field of general surgery and you will undoubtedly be involved in the presentation of these patients during your medical school career and beyond. These include the following:

- Exploratory laparotomy for abdominal pain/bowel obstruction
- Inguinal hernia repair
- Laparoscopic cholecystectomy
- Appendectomy
- Mastectomy
- Colon resection for cancer
- Thyroidectomy/parathyroidectomy
- Coronary artery bypass grafting

Do not miss these cases. Prowl around the ER before you leave to go home, and check the schedule for emergency cases during the day.

Mistake #62

Not seeing trauma surgery

For whatever reason, trauma doesn't occur at times convenient for anyone, so the best way to see trauma is to have your finger on the pulse of the ER. If you can, depending on the system that your program uses, obtain a trauma pager, or work out a deal with your friends on the trauma service to page you when cases arrive in the trauma bay.

Before you leave for the day, look at the operating room schedule to see if there are any add-ons or emergencies scheduled for the evening. The best cases to learn from are the blunt and penetrating traumas that require surgery. These tend to happen when you would least like to be in the hospital, on Friday and Saturday nights, and involve alcohol or other substances … so if you are on call on these nights, make it worth your time and keep an eye on the ER. Introduce yourself to the on-call resident and attending running the trauma service beforehand. When you arrive for the trauma, ask how you can help but stay out of the way for the most part. Once things settle down a bit, you will be asked to help with many aspects of the case, including patient transport, obtaining film reports, and assisting in the operating room.

Mistake **#63**

Not knowing what operations you will be seeing the next day

Before you leave for the day, always check the operating room schedule to see which cases your attending physician(s) will be performing. It is equally important to determine which resident will be scrubbing in on the case since he or she will be teaching you about the case and may even let you open or close.

In general, you are expected to participate in the surgery of all patients you are following. If your patient(s) are not scheduled for surgery, ask your chief resident to assign you a case. It is also reasonable to request a case that you are interested in. Having a case assigned to you the evening before rather than the morning of surgery allows you to prepare adequately for the case, thus maximizing your learning.

Mistake **#64**

Not reading about the case the night before

Reading about the case before the next day's surgery is an absolute must. It is far better to read about the case the evening before rather than the morning of surgery. Reading about the case after you have finished the workday allows for proper preparation. Students who don't adopt this approach may find that the reading time they anticipated they would have in the morning before surgery is not available because patient issues or problems arise, requiring their attention. These students enter the operating room poorly prepared and less knowledgeable about their patient's illness. Their discussion of the case with the surgical attending tends to be more superficial, reflecting the poor grasp they have on the patient's problem and indications for surgery. These students squander a tremendous opportunity to impress the attending.

Mistake **#65**

Not preparing for your attending physician's questions appropriately

At some point during the operation, the attending physician may ask you questions about the case. Students are often afraid that they may be asked questions for which they do not have answers, but attendings do not expect that students will have an answer for every question. It may help to realize that most surgical attendings do not ask questions or "pimp" unless the student has been helpful. Involving you in the discussion and asking you questions means they care about your education. Your job is to answer questions to the best of your ability.

Of course, students who have prepared adequately the evening before surgery are more likely to answer questions appropriately. When preparing for a case, we recommend that you read about your patient's condition, focusing on features of the condition listed in the box below.

For the patient's condition, be prepared to answer questions about the following:

Pathophysiology
Symptoms
Signs
Laboratory testing
Imaging tests
Medical management
Indications for surgery
Timing of surgery
Surgical approaches
Preoperative evaluation
Complications
Outcome
Prognosis
Postoperative management

For cancer operations, be sure to also know the stage and grade of the malignancy.

Success Tip #27
Your preparation the evening before surgery is crucial.

Success Tip #28

Spending a few minutes reviewing important aspects of the disease/surgery just before entering the operating room often proves to be valuable.

Mistake #66

Not knowing what sources to read

The surgery clerkship is not only known for its early starts (sometimes 4 to 4:30 a.m.) but also for its long days. Naturally, students are tired after long days. After arriving home, it's tempting to just relax and call it a day but if you are participating in surgery the next day, you must read about your case. In Mistake # 64, we discussed the importance of reading the evening before surgery. Equally important is using the limited time that you have for preparation wisely and efficiently. We recommend that you focus on four sources for information:

- Start by reading the pages in your basic surgical textbook on the disease process your patient has. The purpose of this source is to master the physiology and learn the indications for surgery.

- Be sure to also use a "high yield" book such as *Surgical Recall* that will focus the information you read in your textbook and highlight the major buzzwords and key surgical points of the case. It will give you an idea of the classic questions that your attending may ask you. This type of book, however, should not be your primary resource.

- A surgical atlas such as *Zollinger's Atlas of Surgical Operations* will provide you with a quick outline of the key maneuvers your surgical team will perform during the case and provide pictures to help you learn the major anatomical landmarks (i.e., the muscles that will be divided, how exposure will be gained, and the major blood vessels and nerves that will be encountered). Using this type of resource will make it easier to stay interested in the case.

● Don't forget that your residents are also a resource. Residents have to prepare for each case and have done so since they were medical students, so they know what is important. They also know what each attending tends to focus on. Many attendings ask the same questions of every student.

Success Tip #29
Don't spend too much time reading about the technical aspects or details of the operative procedure.

Mistake **#67**

Not reviewing the patient's chart before surgery

Before surgery, it is important that you review the patient's chart. Familiarize yourself with the patient's clinical presentation and hospital course. Of course, for inpatients that you have been following, it may not be necessary to review the chart.

If you are assigned or volunteer to participate in the surgery of a patient that is not known to you, you must take the time to review the patient's chart. It's always preferable to review the chart the evening before surgery. Saving the chart review for the morning of the surgery can be problematic, especially if issues related to the care of patients on the floor consume your time.

It may not always be possible to review the chart the evening before surgery. For example, the patient may be having ambulatory surgery and the chart may simply not be available to you. Of course, in this case, you would have no choice but to review it in the morning. If you are planning to review the patient's chart in the morning, be sure to show up in the preoperative holding area before the rest of the team, and certainly before the patient is transported to the operating room.

Mistake #68

Not eating before surgery

It is a good idea to have something for breakfast before scrubbing. Being hungry while in the operating room can certainly distract your focus from the case. Since some surgeries can easily last past lunchtime, if you don't eat, you may develop symptoms of hypoglycemia. Not having breakfast before surgery places you at increased risk of fainting during surgery.

Mistake #69

Leaving valuables in the call room or in the OR locker room

The number of wallets, engagement rings, and watches lost or stolen in the call or OR locker room are too numerous to count. It is best not to bring valuables to the hospital, but if you must, keep these items locked up.

Mistake **#70**

Not going to the bathroom before surgery

This mistake is fairly self-explanatory. Be sure not to drink coffee, tea, soft drinks, or other caffeine-containing products before entering the operating room. Because caffeine has a diuretic effect, its ingestion, especially before a long case, may lead to the need to urinate during surgery.

Mistake **#71**

Not taking your pager off before the case starts

Once you are scrubbed in, you cannot access your beeper. That's why it's important to adopt the system your resident has in place to answer pages when he or she is scrubbed. Often beepers are left with the circulating nurse before you scrub.

Mistake **#72**

Not wearing the proper surgical attire

Proper surgical attire is a must to decrease the patient's risk of developing infection. Without the proper attire, microorganisms present on the skin, clothes, and hair or expelled through the air during breathing or talking might find their way into the patient's deeper tissues which have been exposed by surgery. Proper surgical attire includes:

- Gown
- Gloves
- Caps
- Masks
- Protective eyewear
- Appropriate footwear

Proper surgical attire also decreases your risk of infection. During surgery, operating room personnel may contact or be exposed to potentially infectious bodily fluids, including blood and other tissues. Wearing proper surgical attire reduces this risk.

Mistake #73

Not covering your hair properly

Before entering the surgical suite, be sure that you hair is properly covered. Since hair has a significant bacterial load, it is important to wear a scrub cap or hood that covers all hair surfaces, including sideburns and neckline. If hair is long, a bouffant-style hood or cap should be worn.

Mistake #74

Not wearing your mask appropriately

Before entering the operating room, you must wear a mask. Since breath that escapes from a poorly fitting mask can lead to contamination, you must make sure that you apply the mask properly. It should fit snugly so that your mouth and nose are adequately covered. Consider placing a piece of silk tape across the top edge of the mask to fix the mask to the skin across the bridge of the nose. This simple technique is particularly useful in preventing fogging of the plastic eye shield.

Mistake **#75**

Not protecting your eyes

Sterile team members must wear protective eyewear whenever there is a risk that the patient's bodily fluids may splash into their eyes.

Mistake **#76**

Not wearing appropriate footwear

Since it is common to spend a considerable portion of the day standing in the operating room, it is important to have supportive footwear. Shoes should be sturdy and comfortable. Sandals and other types of open shoes are not acceptable in the operating room environment. Such shoes may slip off or predispose the wearer to a fall, especially with quick movements. Open-type shoes also don't provide the degree of protection that closed shoes offer. The latter offer much more protection in the event that bodily fluids, instruments, or other items fall or come into contact with the feet. Shoes that are worn in the operating room should not be worn outside of the hospital.

Institutional policies regarding shoe covers may vary, but most operating rooms do not require personnel to wear shoe covers. There is no scientific data to suggest that shoe covers reduce the risk of infection. The wearing of shoe covers should be based on the institution's policy as well as the type of surgery being performed. If shoe covers are worn, they must be removed before leaving the operating room suite. Otherwise, blood and other fluids may be introduced to other parts of the department.

Mistake #77

Not following institutional policy regarding the wearing of scrub suits

A two-piece scrub suit, consisting of pant and shirt, is considered proper attire for operating room personnel. According to the Association of Perioperative Registered Nurses (AORN), scrubs should be changed between operations if they become soiled or contaminated. Outside of the OR, policies regarding the wearing of scrubs tend to differ from one institution to another. Be sure to familiarize yourself with the policies at your hospital.

Mistake #78

Not introducing yourself to the operating room team

When you enter the operating room, the first thing you should do (before the patient enters the room or after they fall asleep) is introduce yourself to the scrub nurse, circulating nurse, anesthesiologist, and any surgical assistants. The value of this cannot be underestimated. The operating room team is much more likely to teach and help you if you are polite and respectful.

Write your name on the board so that the circulator can enter it into the operative record and people in the room can refer to you as something other than "the medical student." Pull your own gown/gloves from the storage area and give them to the scrub nurse. The circulator will teach you how to do this in a sterile manner if you ask nicely. The operating room team can help you procure extra sutures or old needle holders after the case to practice with. Your success, comfort, and ability to be in position to assist and observe in the operating room are mainly determined by the OR nurses.

Mistake #79

Not informing the surgical attending or senior resident of a mandatory conference

In many surgery clerkships, there are mandatory lectures. These are lectures that students are required to attend, even if they are in the operating room. Before surgery begins, be sure to let the attending know of the mandatory lecture. Ask him or her what you should do as the time for lectures draws near. Most attendings will simply ask you to remind them 10 or 15 minutes before your lecture starts. They will then allow you to leave for lecture. Before leaving, they may ask you to contact another member of the team to take your place as an assistant.

Mistake **#80**

Scrubbing when your help is needed in the operating room

Before surgery starts, offer to help your resident, circulating nurse, and scrub nurse with any tasks that need to be completed. You may be able to assist in the transfer of the patient to the surgical table, positioning of the patient on the table, placement of the Foley catheter, and preparation of the skin (see Mistake # 81). Your resident will appreciate it if you obtain the necessary films or return phone calls to the floor. For the most part, you should be the last one to gown, and if others are waiting to gown, give them preference (the case can start without you but not without the surgeon).

Success Tip # 30

Well before the operation begins, obtain the patient's radiology films/studies and place them on the viewing board.

Success Tip #31

Don't forget that cases often do not start at their scheduled time. Cases may be cancelled, moved up, or delayed. Keep close watch on the OR board/ schedule. If you notice that a case will be starting sooner than expected, let the student or resident who is expected to participate in the case know so that he or she won't be late.

Mistake **#81**

Not offering to put in the Foley catheter or prep the patient

After the patient is anesthetized, volunteer to place the Foley catheter (if indicated) and prep the patient. If you have questions, ask your resident. If he or she is busy, ask the scrub nurse or circulating nurse for assistance. Learning how to place a Foley catheter is a valuable skill to learn, and it is much easier to gain experience on an anesthetized patient.

The patient's hair around the operative site does not need to be removed before surgery unless its presence interferes with the operation. Razor shaving is no longer recommended because it is associated with higher risk of infection. If hair must be removed, electric clippers should be used right before the operation.

Since the skin is a potential source of microorganisms that may contaminate the wound, the patient's skin needs to be prepped appropriately. This usually involves scrubbing the operative area with an antiseptic solution— the most common being an iodine or chlorhexidine based solution. If you are not sure of the proper technique, ask your resident to show you.

After the skin is prepped, the patient is draped with multiple sterile towels and drapes to expose only the area of interest, and to cover all other areas of the patient and table that the surgeon may encounter. The scrub nurse then sets up at the OR table, sterile light handles are placed on the OR lights, and electrocautery, suction, and other instruments are made available.

To summarize, your role is to help with Foley catheter placement, positioning of the patient, and skin preparation. You may be asked to help with draping once you are scrubbed and sterile.

Success Tip #32
Always volunteer to place the Foley catheter.

Mistake #82

Not asking for help during your first scrub

It's common for students to be unsure of how to scrub when they are first asked to do so. Even though you may have attended the orientation session, there's a difference between hearing about how the scrub is performed and actually having to do it. If you are not sure what to do, don't be afraid to ask your resident for help.

Mistake #83

Not performing the surgical scrub properly

Before donning the sterile gown and gloves, you must perform the surgical scrub. Mistakes students commonly make before or while scrubbing are listed in the following table.

Don't ...	Comment
Forget to remove artificial nails	Artificial nails have been shown to harbor microorganisms
Forget to remove jewelry on your hands or wrists	Microorganisms may be harbored underneath jewelry
Forget to remove necklaces or chains	If necklaces or chains break, they may fall into the wound or otherwise lead to contamination of the sterile field
Use hot water	Antiseptics and soap work much better with warm water
Let water run down your arms in the wrong direction (unscrubbed to scrubbed parts of your arm)	Always keep your hands above the level of your elbow
Scrub for too short a time	A 5-minute scrub is recommended (always scrub for at least as long as the resident and attending surgeon)*
Scrub in a basin with standing water	Standing water predisposes to the growth of microorganisms
Forget to clean under each fingernail	The subungal area contains considerable bacteria
Rinse from the wrong direction	Always rinse the fingertips first
Dry your arm from elbow to fingertips	Always dry the arm from fingertips to elbow
Dry your arms using the same side of the towel	Use a different side of the towel for each arm

Don't ...	Comment
Forget to keep your arms above your waist after you have scrubbed	After scrubbing, your arms should not come into contact with anything until you don your gloves

* A five-minute scrub is recommended for the first scrub of the day; after this three-minute scrubs have been shown to be equivalent to five minute scrubs.

Mistake #84

Not knowing what to do after you scrub

After you scrub, follow the instructions in the order listed below:

- Turn the water off to the scrub sink (but not with your hands!)
- Let the extra water run off your arms into the sink, holding your hands above the level of your elbows, and always above your waist.
- Open the door to the operating room without using your hands/arms (back first)
- Approach the scrub nurse and extend one hand to receive your towel. Wait your turn if your attending or resident is also in the room waiting for a towel. They should be gowned before you.
- Gown and glove
- "Spin" to complete the gowning process
- Help drape if you know how or are asked to help
- Stay out of the way while the setup expeditiously commences

Mistake **#85**

Not knowing where to stand at the OR table

After the resident and attending finish draping the patient, ask the attending where they would like you to stand. Ideally, you should stand where you can see the most, help with retraction, and be in position to suction and cut sutures with good visualization. Try not to stand in between the attending and the scrub nurse. They will be passing sharp instruments to one another and you certainly don't want to be in their path. Do not hesitate to ask for a standing stool if this will help you see (this is an example of where being polite to the circulating nurse pays off).

Mistake **#86**

Not doing your part to maintain the sterile field

All operating room personnel, including scrubbed and nonscrubbed team members, are expected to maintain the sterile field. Within the sterile field are the patient, draped sterile equipment, and other sterile surgical team members. You will observe surgery either as a "sterile" or "nonsterile" team member. "Sterile" team members are those who have scrubbed, gowned, and gloved.

If you are a sterile team member, you must not...

- Leave the sterile field
- Come into contact with any nonsterile object or person
- Reach across unsterile areas
- Touch any item or object below the level of the draped patient
- Fold your arms because the axillary region is not sterile
- Touch your gown below waist level
- Touch your face or back
- Touch the Mayo stand unless the scrub nurse gives you permission

---

If you are a nonsterile (nonscrubbed) team member, you must not...

- Enter the sterile field
- Come into contact with any sterile object or person
- Reach across the sterile sfield
- Touch the Mayo stand

Mistake **#87**

Moving around too much

During surgery, there should be as little movement as possible. This holds true for both scrubbed and nonscrubbed team members. By being aware of where your body is at all times, you will be less likely to make mistakes related to body position or movement.

Scrubbed team members must remain within the sterile area. If you must move, be sure to:

- Pass other sterile team members front to front or back to back
- Face the sterile area as you pass it
- Ask nonsterile team members to step aside rather than try to crowd past them

Nonscrubbed personnel should not move in and out of the surgical suite. This will help prevent dust and bacteria from entering the operating room from the outside. Once inside the operating room, nonscrubbed team members must be aware of their proximity to the sterile field. In general, there should be at least 1 foot of distance between nonsterile team members and the sterile field.

Mistake #88

Not notifying the team if your surgical gloves become contaminated

Sterile team members are expected to wear surgical gloves to protect the patient from microorganisms present on the hands. Gloves also protect operating room personnel from exposure to the patient's potentially infectious bodily fluids and tissues.

You must make every effort to avoid contaminating your surgical gloves. Gloves may become contaminated because you inadvertently touch your hand to your face or other part of your body or clothing that is not sterile. Dropping one or both of your gloved hands below the level of your waist is also considered contamination. The box below provides information on what to do should your surgical gloves become contaminated.

If your surgical gloves become contaminated, you should...

1. Stop your activity
2. Step away from the sterile field
3. Take off the contaminated glove
4. Put on new gloves (if your hands are soiled by the patient's bodily fluids, you must perform a surgical scrub before putting on new gloves)

Students often do not realize that they have contaminated their surgical gloves. The contamination often comes to light when another team member notices a breach in aseptic technique. Sometimes no one else realizes that contamination has taken place other than student. In these cases, it is important that students let the team know. Students are often tempted not to disclose this to the team for fear of embarrassment or rebuke but this, of course, is not in the best interests of the patient or themselves.

Mistake #89

Arguing with the scrub nurse or surgeon when they say you are contaminated

Scrubbed medical students in the operating room for the first time will often unknowingly touch something that is not sterile. If someone notices that you are contaminated, do not argue even if you don't agree. Simply nod your head and change whatever is now contaminated.

Mistake **#90**

Not involving yourself in the case

The team is more apt to teach and involve you in a case if you show some interest and initiative. Always ask to scrub in for a case. Ask intelligent questions. Offer to hold retractors, cut sutures, and provide suction. While these initial efforts are certainly important, it is also essential to maintain your interest and focus throughout the entire surgery. It is very easy to become tired or let your mind wander off, especially when you are involved in longer cases. You must guard against losing focus while in the operating room to avoid looking uninterested in the case. If you stay focused, there is a good chance that you will get to do more, such as closing the incision.

Mistake **#91**

Being discouraged if the surgeon is giving you a hard time or "pimping" you

There are often tense moments during an operation, and the difference between a good and bad outcome can be determined in seconds. Things move fast and perfect execution is demanded…often there is not time for pleasantries.

You need to have thick skin in the operating room; do what you are told but nothing more, and stay focused on the task at hand. If you are not helpful in the operating room, you will not be given any role in the case. That's why it's important to make adjustments without losing

99

your cool and keep perspective on your interactions. By exhibiting emotional intelligence in the operating room, you will be given greater involvement in the case.

Success Tip #33

Surgeons don't pimp students to embarrass or humiliate them. It is a teaching technique. Once you fully realize this, your experience will be more positive.

Success Tip #34

Don't view pimping as something to be feared or avoided. Instead, view it as an opportunity to shine. Embrace pimp sessions.

Success Tip #35

If your fellow student or resident is struggling to answer a question, do not jump in and answer the question.

Mistake #92

Not answering the question you were asked

Most questions are asked quickly in the operating room. Because the attending physician who asked you the question is already thinking of the next move in the surgery, answer the question succinctly. If you do not know the answer, there is only one acceptable response, "I do not know, but I will find out before the end of the day." The next time you are with that attending, thank them for highlighting the importance of the question and let them know that you did in fact look it up.

Mistake **#93**

Asking a question at an inappropriate time of the case

Questions are encouraged and necessary, but only at the appropriate time. You do not want to distract the surgeon when he or she is actively performing a task or in a complicated portion of the case. If you think of the surgery as a classical music piece, there are times of adagio, allegro, crescendo, and decrescendo. Try to look for the adagio portions of the case, when things are moving smoothly and the team is dissecting in a relatively safe area, not precariously navigating around nerves and vessels. Even if your question demonstrates amazing insight and profound interest, it will not be perceived as such if it is asked at a delicate time. Assessment of your performance is partly based on your operating room maturity level, and learning when to ask questions is one of the best measures of this.

Success Tip #36

You should not feel foolish asking questions. Asking questions shows the surgeon your enthusiasm, interest, and energy.

Success Tip #37

Before asking a question, always ask the surgeon if it's a good time to do so.

Mistake #94

Not understanding the attending or resident physician's request

As a member of the surgical team, you need to realize that your contributions are important to the success of the surgery. During the operation, the resident or attending may ask you to retract, tie knots, or cut sutures. If you didn't hear what was said, don't understand something that is asked of you, or are not sure how to proceed, don't be afraid to ask for clarification or reiteration of the instructions.

Mistake #95

Not retracting properly

Retracting is arguably the most important and most difficult job in the operating room. Proper exposure of the field of interest is paramount to a successful surgery, and armed with a retractor, this is your mission. The attending will most likely choose the correct retractor for you and put it in the correct place with appropriate tension. Mimic this exactly and hold it steady, but be aware of what is going on and try to adjust accordingly with the surgeon's permission. Do not move unless told to—you may be exposing a vessel or structure that you cannot see.

It is common for students to lighten up on their retracting with time as their hand fatigues but this may lead to the retractor slipping out of its assigned location. To avoid this, rest your hand by placing another hand below it or switch hands, if possible.

Keep in mind that pulling too hard can cause tissue damage, ischemia, and nerve damage. Also remember not to lean on the patient when holding the retractor. This can be difficult when you are standing sideways, can't see what you are exposing, and playing twister with the surgeon next to you for an hour, but you can hurt the patient by leaning on him. For example, leaning on the leg, chest, and face can cause distal ischemia, inhibit ventilation, and dislodge the endotracheal tube, respectively.

Mistake #96

Not cutting the sutures the correct length

Different attendings have different preferences, but as a general rule of thumb, think of sutures in two categories: monofilament (e.g., prolene/monocryl) and multifilament (e.g., vicryl/silk). Monofilament sutures are more "slippery," so as a security measure, the tails are cut a little longer—about 1 cm. Multifilament sutures can be cut about 2-3 mm above the knot. Ultimately, the correct length of a suture is whatever the attending prefers. Always ask how long the ends of a suture should be the first time you cut that particular suture type. Then proceed to cut the remaining sutures of the same type to the length specified. Cut both tails at the same time with the tips of the scissors and pull away gently. If the suture is incompletely cut, pulling away too fast could undo the knot. Always use the very tip of the scissors for cutting to minimize the risk of inadvertently cutting something behind the suture. If you are not told otherwise after a few snips, you are likely doing a good job.

Mistake #97

Loud talking or socializing in the operating room

Though the attending may have music playing and others in the room may be talking, once the incision is made, you must stay focused on the task at hand. Socializing or loud talking during the case can be a distraction to the surgeon and is considered poor operating room etiquette. This tends to be more of a problem for nonscrubbed students, who may hold private conversations with other students. This, of course, can affect the surgeon's concentration and will undoubtedly upset him.

Mistake #98

Paging the resident when he or she is in the operating room

If you need to contact your resident, do not page the resident when he or she is in the operating room, unless it is essential. Beeping the resident while he or she is operating is distracting and a waste of operating room resources. Remember that someone on the operating room team will have to answer the page when the beeper rings. If an issue arises that requires urgent attention, contact a resident who is not in the operating room. Typically, a junior surgical resident is available to handle issues that arise while the rest of the team is operating.

Mistake **#99**

Not offering to answer the resident or attending physician's pager

If you are a nonscrubbed observer, offer to answer the resident or attending's pager should it beep. Your offer may or may not be accepted but it will certainly be appreciated. If it is accepted, you will have an opportunity to relieve a member of the operating team (usually the circulator) of a responsibility that, at times, can interrupt the flow of surgery.

Mistake **#100**

Not knowing what to do if you feel faint

If you do feel faint during surgery, notify the other sterile team members as soon as possible. Sometimes students don't let the team know about how they are feeling, only to faint forward, contaminating the sterile field. Their reluctance to inform the team of an impending faint often has to do with fear that they will look foolish. Remember that everyone who has worked in the operating room has felt faint or ill at some point. By letting the team know, actions can be taken to prevent harm from occurring to either the patient or yourself. Simply let the team know, ask to step back, and scrub out. If you cannot avoid falling, remember to always fall backwards.

Mistake #101

Not knowing what to do when you have to sneeze

If you have to sneeze while scrubbed, back your head away from the surgical field, steady yourself, and sneeze straight into your mask. Turning your head to the side exposes the only open part of your mask to the sterile field.

Mistake #102

Not writing the operative note immediately

The operative note serves many purposes:

- It helps you summarize the surgery, and when done repeatedly for many different surgeries, gives you a better idea of the indications, pathology, fluid requirements, blood loss, and important operative findings for each case.

- It allows you to interact with the anesthesia team and to know about their concerns and role in the case.

- It gives you a role at the end of the case that, if done well, helps make you appear dependable, trustworthy, and responsible.

Write the note while the patient is being awakened. When the resident is not otherwise occupied, have him or her read your note and cosign it before you drop off the patient in the post-anesthesia care unit (PACU).

Commonly made mistakes on the operative note are discussed in Chapter 4.

Success Tip #38

At the end of the case, grab the chart and begin writing the operative note. Don't wait for your resident to ask you to do so.

Mistake **#103**

Not accompanying the patient to the Post-Anesthesia Care Unit (PACU)

Always help transfer the patient to a gurney after the case and accompany the team to the PACU. Manpower is needed to move the patient and an extra hand may be needed to help wheel the gurney. In addition to accompanying the patient to the PACU, participate in your patient's care there.

Mistake **#104**

Not seeing the patient whose surgery you took part in before afternoon rounds and before going home

Always check on your patient in the PACU and again on the floor. It's never good if your patient had a complication 30 minutes after surgery and you did not know about it until the afternoon or the next morning. Visit your patient in the PACU and again on the floor either before afternoon rounds or before you go home if it was a late case. Write a postoperative note on your patient a few hours after surgery. Commonly made mistakes on the postoperative note are discussed in Chapter 5.

Mistake #105

Not familiarizing yourself with knot tying and suture techniques early in the rotation

Early in the surgery rotation, familiarize yourself with knot tying and basic sutures such as running, subcuticular, vertical mattress, and horizontal mattress stitches. Often there will be a suture course for students to attend. Keep an eye out for these courses even when you are on other rotations. Also ask your resident to show you these basic techniques. Once you have been introduced to them, practice these techniques so that you are ready to perform them in the operating room. You should have a packet of sutures on you at all times and practice knots whenever you have down time - between cases, etc. If you know how to tie a basic knot and do a subcuticular suture, your resident will often let you tie sutures along the way and close the incision. It is a great way to show you are interested and be involved in the case.

Success Tip #39
Practice tying knots outside the operating room. This practice will come in handy in the event that you are given the opportunity to tie knots or place sutures.

Attending Interactions

Surgery attending rounds at many institutions, unlike medicine attending rounds, may be 5-10 minutes per day or even non-existent. Depending on whether you do your surgical rotation at a private or public hospital, your interaction with the attending during clinic may also be limited. Most medical students will spend the bulk of their time with the attending in the operating room. Since most of your interactions with attending physicians will take place in the operating room, the overall impression you make on the attending physician will largely be based on your verbal and nonverbal communication during surgery. In this chapter, we discuss mistakes students commonly make in their interactions with attending physicians.

Mistake **#106**

Not asking other students or residents about your attending

All surgeons are impressed with students who not only perform thorough patient evaluations but also display enthusiasm, interest, and a strong fund of knowledge. Of course, there are many other qualities that attending physicians place a high value on. For example, it is expected that students conduct themselves with the highest degree of professionalism in their relations with health care professionals and patients. What is often less apparent to students is the degree of importance that an individual attending physician may place on certain qualities or skills. Students are also unsure of an attending physician's tendencies or preferences, especially early in the rotation. Usually, through a process of trial and error, what the attending physician is looking for and what he or she considers important becomes clear. The initial period of uncertainty, discomfort, and awkwardness can be lessened if students ask other students or residents, who have worked with the attending physician, about preferences and expectations.

Mistake #107

Not showing initiative

Attending surgeons (and residents) are very impressed with students who show initiative. Students who begin or complete tasks without prompting from their superiors are showing initiative. Examples include:

- Volunteering to help perform a bedside procedure rather than waiting to be asked by the resident or attending physician

- Looking up relevant literature on your own when the team is not sure how to proceed with a difficult management problem

Before tackling issues and problems on your own, it's preferable to ask your attending physician if he or she would like you to begin or complete a task, especially if you are not sure of how the attending prefers to have these tasks completed. For example, attending physicians may be upset if a student pulls out a drain before being told.

Mistake #108

Not being confident

Attending physicians are much more impressed by a student able to answer questions with confidence. The best way to become confident, of course, is to read about your patient's condition and practice your answers to anticipated questions.

Mistake #109

Not answering questions appropriately

In speaking with attending physicians, you should be succinct and to the point. Long, drawn-out answers to a pimp question or a question about a patient's condition are not appreciated. A few pet peeves of surgeons to avoid when being pimped:

- Never answer a question with a question – "Ummm…is it the Triangle of Calot?" See Mistake #108.

- Never say, "I don't know" immediately. At least try to make an educated guess before you say, "I don't know the answer to that question, but I'll look it up and tell you tomorrow."

- Don't give a long-winded answer to the question or answer a question that was not asked. Be succinct.

To prepare for pimping, see Mistake #65.

Mistake #110

Not asking questions appropriately

Surgeons love when students ask questions because it is an indication of interest in the field. In the operating room and during rounds, however, there is a right and wrong time to ask a question (see Mistake #93). As a general rule, if no one else is talking during the case, you probably shouldn't either.

Despite what your grade school teachers told you, however, there are dumb questions. Try not to ask obvious questions like, "Is that the gallbladder?" Your attending expects a basic knowledge of anatomy and pathology; never ask questions about things you could easily look up in a medical student textbook. Rather, surgeons are impressed by insightful questions such as, "What are the advantages of repairing an inguinal hernia with a synthetic mesh over a Bassini Repair?"

Invariably, attending physicians will ask if you have any questions. It is in your best interest to read enough about the case or patient to ask a few intelligent questions; "No, I don't" is not an acceptable answer. Most importantly, be sincere in your curiosity. Surgeons often see through students who ask questions because they think it will help their grade.

On Call

The term "call" refers to a period of time during which your team is accepting new patient admissions and is responsible for the evaluation of issues or problems that arise in already hospitalized patients. Typically, a student will be on call with one or more residents on the team. Together, you will tackle the challenges of the on call experience. While being on call often elicits anxiety in students, it can be an exhilarating experience, one that offers you tremendous learning opportunities. In this chapter, we will discuss commonly made mistakes while on call.

Mistake **#111**

Complaining about the call schedule

At some institutions, the call schedule may be created well before you arrive on the rotation. If you know of a personal obligation that would make it difficult for you to take call on a particular day, be sure to notify whoever creates the schedule well before the rotation starts so that your needs can be met. The individual who creates the student call schedule may vary from one place to another but may include the clerkship director, departmental secretary, or chief surgical resident. If you are scheduled to be on call when you need to be away for personal reasons (i.e., wedding of sister, etc.), do not complain to the creator of the call schedule. Instead, do everything you can to correct the problem yourself. If switching is allowed, approach one of your classmates to see if he or she would like to trade calls. This approach is much better than complaining about the schedule to your team members. In addition, avoid complaining about the number of call nights you have been assigned, weekend call duties, and any perceived inequality between your call schedule and that of other students.

Mistake #112

Being unfamiliar with on-call responsibilities

The anxiety associated with being on call can be lessened if you are aware of your responsibilities. Your responsibilities include, but are not limited to, those listed below.

Student responsibilities while on call
Writing preoperative notes
Writing postoperative notes
Evaluating new patient admissions from the ER
Evaluating problems that arise in hospitalized patients
Evaluating newly arrived trauma patients
Recording the new patient's H & P
Drawing blood
Changing wound dressings
Pulling tubes/drains
Performing procedures
Scrubbing in and assisting on any operative procedures
Participating in codes

At the start of your first call, meet with the on-call resident to learn about his or her expectations for you. If you happen to work with different residents on subsequent calls, be sure to have the same discussion since expectations vary from one resident to another. In other words, what worked well for you with one resident may not serve you well with another.

You also want to learn about tasks that need to be completed. Quite often, the surgery resident will already have a list of things to do. He or she may assign you some of these tasks or you may tackle them together. Be sure that you inform the resident of how he or she can reach you.

Mistake **#113**

Being unenthusiastic

The on call experience can be physically demanding and exhausting. The initial enthusiasm and energy that you brought to the start of call might be tempered as the number of patients assigned to you increases, tasks to be completed multiply, and the effects of fatigue or sleep deprivation sets in. Despite the obstacles in your way, remain enthusiastic. Your resident will certainly notice your positive attitude and will reward your interest, enthusiasm, and assistance with increased teaching and opportunities to participate in or perform various procedures. Your efforts may also result in an increased role in the operating room later in the rotation.

Mistake #114

Missing out on the action

A common behavior of medical students on call is to tell the resident to page him or her when there is something going on. They then retire to the student call room or the library, getting a page or two during the night when major developments occur (i.e., new patient admission). When paged, respond to the page quickly because if you are difficult to reach, the resident will not spend further time searching for you.

While you may certainly adopt this approach, instead of retiring to the call room or library, we recommend that you tag along with the on call resident (if he or she does not mind). By doing so, you will be involved in not just the major developments but also the minor ones, all of which can present you with unique learning opportunities. If you don't accompany the resident, the resident will find it easier to do something on his or her own rather than page you in the call-room, wait for you to call back, tell you what to do, how to do it, and then check to make sure it's done.

By tagging along with the resident, you will be able to see what kind of responsibilities he or she has on-call. By observing, you may become familiar with many of the skills you will need when you are a house officer. If you establish yourself as honest, dependable, and hardworking, you will be given tasks that will grow more interesting and more challenging (e.g., central lines, laceration repairs, or even chest tubes).

Furthermore, you'll be present to see the emergencies that the on-call resident wouldn't otherwise have time to tell you about, such as cardiac arrests or bedside cricothyroidotomies and thoracotomies.

Mistake **#115**

Not seeking ways to help

General offerings of help (i.e. "Let me know how I can help") are nice, but there are even better ways to impress the resident. When on call, a resident has plenty of other things to worry about. Making sure you are not bored is not one of them. Indeed, unless the resident is familiar with your work, he or she may think it is easier to just do the work alone. You have to make *specific* offers to help.

For example, let's say that you just saw a consult in the ER with the on-call resident. The resident grabs the chart before you are able to and starts looking for a blank page to write a consult note. Instead of watching him write the note, say, "I can write the note while you write the orders," or "I'll get some supplies for the procedure while you are writing the note."

Why is this important? The ultimate purpose of proactively, sometimes aggressively, offering help is not just to allow the resident to get to bed earlier (though this would surely be appreciated). You are doing this to gain experience in doing the things that you will do as an intern or resident (a role that you may have in as little as 12 months). Such tasks may include writing orders, evaluating patients, or increasing your efficiency at obtaining the information necessary for a thorough history and physical.

Taking this type of initiative will help you impress the resident as an autonomous, dependable, and enthusiastic medical student. Because these are some of the qualities that surgery residents and attending physicians value, this type of effort will likely lead to a rewarding clerkship evaluation.

Mistake **#116**

Not writing preoperative and postoperative notes

During call, preoperative notes should be written for patients undergoing surgery the next day. For patients who have had surgery that day, postoperative notes should be written. If they were already written, check on the patient in their room. It is expected that you will write preoperative and postoperative notes on patients you are following. You should also offer to write preoperative and postoperative notes for other patients on the service. Your help can ease the workload on your busy surgical resident. Please refer to the chapters on preoperative and postoperative note writing for further information.

Mistake **#117**

Not going the full distance with the evaluation and management of a new patient

While on call, you will be responsible for evaluating newly hospitalized patients. The patients that you pick up will be yours for the duration of their hospital stay. It is a wonderful opportunity to be involved in the patient's care from the beginning to the end of the hospitalization, including any operative intervention the patient may require.

Typically, these patients will be admitted to the hospital through the emergency room. Your initial contact with the patient may be in the emergency room or after arrival to the hospital ward. Your responsibilities for the evaluation and management of a newly admitted patient are as follows:

- Obtain the patient's history
- Perform the physical examination
- Gather laboratory test data
- Gather imaging test data
- Analyze information and develop assessment and plan
- Present the patient to your resident
- Write admit orders
- Write the H & P

With every new patient assigned to you, strive to function as much as possible as the patient's intern.

Mistake #118

Not obtaining a complete history on newly admitted patients

As a student, it is expected that you will obtain a complete history. A complete history includes the information listed below.

Elements of the complete history
Source of history
Reliability of source
Chief complaint
History of present illness
Past medical history
Past surgical history
Medications (name, dose, frequency, route of administration)
Allergies (along with manifestations of the drug allergy)
Social history (including tobacco, alcohol, and drug use)
Family history

Review of systems:

General	Genitourinary
Skin	Gynecological
Eyes	Neurological
Ears	Psychiatric
Nose/throat	Hematologic
Cardiac	Musculoskeletal
Respiratory	Endocrine
Gastrointestinal	

Mistake #119

Not performing a complete physical examination on newly admitted patients

Physical examinations performed by students are expected to be complete. Following are the elements of the complete physical examination.

Elements of the complete physical examination

General appearance
Vital signs (temperature, pulse, respirations,
    blood pressure, height, weight)
Skin
Lymph nodes
Head
    General
    Eyes
    Ears
    Nose
    Mouth (teeth, tongue, throat)
Neck (including thyroid)
Thorax
Breast
Cardiovascular (including heart and pulses)
Pulmonary
Abdomen
Genitourinary
Rectal
Extremity
Back
Neurological
    Level of consciousness
    Orientation
    Sensory/motor function
    Cerebellar function

One of your chief responsibilities as a medical student is obtaining and performing a complete history and physical examination on newly admitted patients. After doing so, it is necessary to carefully consider the information you have collected. It is this information that is used to determine what the patient's likely diagnosis is among a list of possibilities known as the differential diagnosis. It is said that 80 to 90% of diagnoses can be established after the history and physical examination. Too often, students don't give enough thought to the clinical significance of the findings elicited in the history and physical examination. Instead, too much emphasis is placed on laboratory, imaging, and other sophisticated testing. While this testing certainly has an important role in the evaluation of these patients, do not forget that the money is in the history and physical examination.

Mistake #120

Not gathering the laboratory/ imaging test data

Laboratory and imaging tests are generally performed to confirm or exclude a diagnosis that is suggested by the patient's clinical presentation. They may also be obtained to follow the course of an established disease. Any abnormality that is identified should be interpreted in the context of the patient's clinical presentation. In the following box, we have highlighted the differences between the average and star student in the area of laboratory test interpretation.

The average student …	The star student …
Gathers laboratory/ imaging test data	Gathers laboratory/ imaging test data
Views the imaging/ pathology test with the resident	Views the imaging/ pathology tests on their own and then with the resident Obtains the official reading from the radiologist/ pathologist

The average student …	The star student …
Identifies abnormalities	Identifies abnormalities Understands the clinical significance of the abnormalities or looks them up Understands the rationale for ordering the tests Recognizes the need for further testing to confirm the diagnosis and makes sure the testing is performed (draws blood or transports patient for test, if necessary) Relays the test results back to the resident (brings the film or study to the resident if necessary) Develops an approach to elucidating the etiology of unexplained abnormalities

Mistake #121

Not understanding the treatment plan

Formulate the treatment plan on your own. Then discuss it with the resident. In your plan, be sure to address the following questions.

Questions to address in the treatment plan

Is conservative (medical) rather than operative treatment appropriate?

If medical treatment is appropriate, what treatment is considered the standard of care (observation, intravenous fluids, antibiotics, analgesic therapy, etc.)?

If an operation is needed, does it need to be performed immediately or later that night?

Can the patient be discharged (for ER consults)?

If you simply present the patient information without providing your thoughts regarding the patient's management, your resident will certainly fill in the blanks. When you don't independently formulate a treatment plan, you lose out on a valuable opportunity to practice clinical reasoning. The ability to develop a sound plan is not an innate skill but one that becomes more refined with knowledge, practice, and experience.

When you have decided on the treatment plan, be sure that you have a solid understanding of the treatment plan. In the following table, we have described the characteristics that differentiate the star student from the average student with regards to the treatment plan.

The average student …	The star student …
Develops a treatment plan	Develops a treatment plan independently and then discusses it with the resident Understands the rationale behind the plan Considers how the treatment may affect the patient's other medical problems Follows through to make sure the patient receives the treatment Is familiar with the adverse effects of the therapy Understands the indications for operative intervention

Mistake #122

Not writing the admission orders

You should write the admission orders on every new patient assigned to you. Here's an area where you need to be aggressive because if you don't volunteer to write the orders, then your resident will take care of it on his or her own.

Nurses and other healthcare professionals rely on the admission orders to provide the care needed for the patient and his or her medical problems. What is ordered will vary from patient to patient depending on the patient's conditions. However, the components of each patient's admission orders are the same. By using the mnemonic ABC VANDALISM, the student can be confident that all the components or elements of the admission orders will be included.

Mnemonic for admission orders
Date and time
Admit to **B**ecause (diagnosis) **C**ondition **V**ital signs **A**ctivity **N**ursing **D**iet **A**llergies **L**aboratory tests **I**V orders **S**pecial orders **M**edications
Signature/name

As an example, consider a 30-year old man who will be admitted from the ER for observation. He was the passenger in a car involved in a frontal-impact motor vehicle accident. Upon admission, he was awake and alert. His only complaint was mild generalized abdominal pain. Physical examination reveals only minimal tenderness but no signs of peritonitis. Although a CT scan of his abdomen showed no abnormalities, he will be admitted overnight for observation (often done to rule out small bowel injury, an injury that is often not seen on a CT scan). The admission orders for this patient are listed in the following table.

01/01/04
18:35

Admit to: Trauma Surgery A Service (Dr. Jones), ward 5B

Diagnosis: Abdominal pain s/p MVA

Condition: Fair

Vitals: BP, P, RR, SpO_2, temp q 8 hours.

Activity: As tolerated

Nursing: Please record strict inputs and outputs
Head of bed at 30 degrees
Notify house officer for:
- temperature >100.5°C
- P>100 or <60
- SBP>150 or <100
- DBP>100 or <60.
- respiratory rate >25 or <15
- urine output <30 mL/hour

Diet: Clear liquid diet

Allergies: NKDA

Labs: CBC c platelets, serum biochemistries in AM

IV orders: Heplock

Special orders: TED hose and SCDs to both legs while in bed

Medications: None

Ted Williams, MS-3 /

In the following table, we have described the characteristics that differentiate the star student from the average student regarding the writing of the admission order.

The average student ...	The star student ...
Lets the resident write admission orders	Takes the initiative to write the admission orders Discusses the orders with the resident Understands the rationale behind the orders written Follows through to make sure that the orders are carried out

Mistake #123

Not relaying information accurately

While a good deal of paperwork and many procedures are involved, most of the work done by a resident on call is spent gathering, analyzing, and relaying information. After a new patient is admitted, for example, defining a plan of care often takes only 30 minutes. Following up on blood tests that were ordered, radiologist readings of a CT scan, consultant input, and other information sources, on the other hand, often consumes much more time. You may be of most benefit to your team or the on-call resident by obtaining and accurately relaying certain information. Check the computer regularly for expected lab test results. Check on the patient in his or her room to see if the radiology tech has come by for the follow-up portable chest x-ray. Follow-up on things which have been set in motion earlier in the day or evening.

Doing some of this "legwork" for the on-call resident will often result in the more enjoyable rewards— placing a chest tube, suturing a laceration, or putting in a central line. You will also learn a great deal of medicine while establishing yourself as hardworking and dependable, qualities that faculty and residents often focus on when writing an evaluation.

Mistake **#124**

Not taking advantages of opportunities in the SICU

In the Surgical Intensive Care Unit or SICU, procedures are commonly performed throughout the day. When you become an intern or resident, you will be asked to perform these procedures. Observing and participating in procedures as a student will help prepare you for that time.

If your call team is covering the SICU, it may be your resident who is asked to perform these procedures. If so, help your resident with them. If coverage of the SICU is not the responsibility of your team, you may still be allowed to help with these procedures if you introduce yourself to the SICU resident and express an interest in participating.

Do not forget about your other clinical responsibilities, which, of course, take precedence. Your resident will not be pleased if tasks assigned to you are delayed or not completed because you decided to spend time in the SICU. To avoid this situation from happening, always touch base with your resident, seek his or her permission, and avoid asking when things are busy for your team.

Mistake #125

Not participating in the evaluation and surgery of trauma patients

Trauma patients generally present to the emergency room. They may or may not be admitted to your team. Even if they are not admitted to your team, be sure to involve yourself in these cases from initial evaluation to management, including any operative intervention. Participation in the care of these patients not only provides you with a valuable learning experience but it will also help prepare you for examination questions. Trauma questions are common on the surgery shelf examination, and your experience evaluating and managing trauma patients will help you answer these questions correctly.

Commonly Made Mistakes on the

Surgical Oral Examination

In addition to a written examination, many surgery clerkships require their students to take an oral examination at the end of the rotation. Most students have little if any experience with this examination format. The ability to perform well on the oral examination is based not only on a strong foundation of basic surgical principles but a combined ability to communicate the appropriate evaluation and treatment of a theoretical patient. The goal of this chapter is to examine the role of the student and proctor during the examination process to eliminate potential errors before and during examination.

Before the Examination

Mistake **#126**

Not being prepared for the examination

An oral examination is unique in that there are no answers to choose from on a piece of paper. Therefore, appropriate preparation is essential before entering the room. However, since surgery is such a large subject, it is in your best interests to focus your time on common surgical problems (e.g., electrolyte abnormalities, cholecystitis, breast cancer, bowel obstruction, diverticulitits) encountered on a regular basis. Remember that the proctor does not expect you to know the entire textbook of surgery; thus, concentrate on high-yield topics (see also Mistake #128).

Mistake **#127**

Not knowing the format of the oral examination early in the rotation

While an oral examination can be administered in several different formats, most commonly, surgery clerkships will employ a cognitive format. In this format, the student is given a brief clinical scenario and is allowed to ask the examiner pertinent questions about that scenario. The student may ask the examiner questions about the patient's history and physical examination, may be asked to develop a differential diagnosis, can ask for relevant laboratory and imaging test results, and uses the information given to establish a diagnosis and formulate a treatment plan. A less commonly used format is the clinical format, in which the student presents and discusses a patient he or she worked up during the rotation ("a known case").

It is important for you to be aware of the oral examination format used in your clerkship. Once you know of the format, you will be better able to study and prepare for what you will encounter. The cognitive oral examination format tends to be favored in most surgery clerkships. Examiners are often, but not always, given a list of cases or clinical scenarios from which to choose. Generally, two or three scenarios are presented to the student and the evaluation of the student's performance is based on the reasoning skills and clinical judgement that the student demonstrates. In the remainder of this chapter, we will discuss mistakes that commonly occur before and during a cognitive oral examination.

Mistake **#128**

Not knowing what topics to prepare for

While the list of cases (clinical scenarios) may not be shared with students, when the information is made known to students, it certainly makes preparation for the examination easier. If the list of cases is not available to you, you should ask residents and faculty what they consider high yield topics. Don't forget to ask students in your class (or in the class above you if this is the first rotation of the academic year) who have already completed the clerkship about the topics that they encountered on the oral examination.

Following, we have listed some common patient scenarios that may be presented to you during the examination. In your preparation for the examination, think carefully about how you would evaluate such patients. During the examination, you will be expected to ask the examiner for information such as more history, a physical examination, lab testing, etc. that will help you not only establish the diagnosis but also develop a management plan.

Sample Study Questions

1. 55-year old female presents with a palpable left breast mass.
2. 22-year old female presents with a palpable thyroid nodule.
3. 75-year old male with constipation and a change in the caliber of his stools.
4. 25-year old male with right lower quadrant pain.
5. 47-year old female with right upper quadrant pain.

6. 65-year old male with left lower quadrant pain.

7. 55-year old male with previous abdominal surgery now presents with partial small bowel obstruction. What electrolytes abnormalities would you expect?

8. 45-year old female with history of alcohol abuse presents with epigastric/right upper quadrant pain.

9. 75-year old male with history of atrial fibrillation now presents with abdominal pain out of proportion to the physical examination.

10. 67-year old male with significant smoking history presents with increasing right leg pain with ambulation.

11. 60-year old male with significant smoking history presents with episodes of transient blindness.

12. 16-year old asymptomatic female with elevated serum calcium levels on routine screening laboratories on yearly high school physical.

13. 64-year old male presents with nausea/vomiting and abdominal distension.

14. 53-year old male with microcytic anemia and dizziness.

15. 16-year old female presents with gun shot wound to left upper quadrant.

16. 22-year old male status post motor vehicle accident presents with altered mental status.

17. 17-year old male status post posterior knee dislocation presents with cold distal extremity.

18. 22-year old male status post crush injury to the right lower extremity now with loss of distal sensation.

19. 70-year old male presents with a 7 cm abdominal aortic aneurysm.

20. 65-year old male who, on preoperative chest x-ray for right inguinal hernia repair, is found to have a solitary pulmonary nodule.

You will encounter some of the clinical scenarios above in patients that are assigned to you during the clerkship. It is important to understand that, in a two- or three-month clerkship, it will be difficult to see all clinical scenarios you might be asked about during an oral examination. For this reason, you will want to keep your eyes and ears open, making a concerted effort to learn about patients on the service in whose care you are not directly participating. Make every effort to attend clerkship lectures because questions on the examination may come from topics that are covered in the lecture series.

Mistake **#129**

Not understanding the grading process

To administer an oral examination to so many students at the end of a clerkship, a number of faculty members are needed to serve as proctors. In your interactions with faculty, you have undoubtedly come across some that are more difficult to please and others that are not as hard to impress. With that said, you may be concerned that you might be assigned to a more demanding grader while your fellow student is assigned to a less demanding grader. You may wonder how fair such a test may be.

Because faculty expectations vary regarding the depth of knowledge a third year medical student should have, many clerkships have tried to standardize their oral examination by educating faculty on what are considered appropriate responses (e.g., knowledge level) for a third year medical student. Examiners may be given an evaluation form with a checklist of items. For example, if a student asks questions to elicit relevant information from the history, a check may be placed in the corresponding box. Another check may be placed if the student selects appropriate diagnostic tests and so on. At the end of the examination, the examiner can add up the point values of boxes that have been checked to yield a cumulative score. Such an approach helps examiners grade a student's performance more objectively.

Mistake #130

Assuming that you will easily be able to express your thoughts

During the examination, one of the hardest things to do is to express your thoughts in a logical manner. Think back to the first time you presented a patient. Unless you took the time and effort to practice your presentation, you were very disorganized and hard to follow. The same holds true for your oral examination; it takes practice to look and perform your best. Therefore, performing mock oral examinations with your friends is an invaluable experience prior to the actual examination. When taking an oral examination, verbalize every action; non-verbalization means the action did not occur. For example, all physicians perform an ABC (airway, breathing, circulation) assessment on each patient but typically do not verbalize it. However, on an oral examination, not stating the ABCs is comparable to not performing the ABCs. Don't assume the proctor can or will read your mind.

Mistake #131

Not considering the importance of your presentation

The worst thing to allow prior to the initiation of the examination is the stereotyping of yourself as an improper student. In the ideal world, this should not happen, but the best solution is to eliminate the possibility. Your goal is to portray a calm and professional attitude at the beginning of the examination. Therefore, dress appropriately (business casual), arrive early (30 minutes prior to the examination), and be cordial and respectful. While your appearance, behavior, and manners will not guarantee an outstanding performance, they can certainly help you create a positive impression, one that you can build upon. Do not underestimate the importance of establishing the right professional presence.

Mistake #132

Not having a strategy for the oral examination

As you prepare for the oral examination, you will want to develop a strategy that enables you to show the examiner that you can logically evaluate the clinical scenario that is presented to you, covering all the areas that are expected. We recommend starting with the mnemonic, AIDE, which is described below.

Using AIDE

Step 1: Assess ABCs – airway, breathing, and circulation – in every patient

Step 2: Institute differential diagnosis. Offer the examiner a list of potential causes for the patient's clinical presentation based on the information already given.

Step 3: Determine relevant positives and negative from the history and physical examination. In other words, ask the examiner for key information that will help you narrow the differential diagnosis to the most likely diagnosis.

Step 4: Establish appropriate radiographic and/or laboratories tests (only if needed) to be ordered. Tests may be needed to confirm the diagnosis, exclude other possibilities, and assess the severity of the illness.

For patients who have indications for surgery, once you have established the diagnosis using the AIDE mnemonic, use the mnemonic PIP to make sure you cover important aspects of preoperative, intraoperative, and postoperative care.

Using PIP

Step 1: Pre-operative assessment
- Does the patient have any comorbidities? (i.e. CAD, CVA, COPD, hepatic insufficiency)? If so, can they be optimized?
- Does the patient need resuscitation?
- Does the patient need correction of electrolytes?
- Does the patient need neo-adjuvant chemotherapy (if the preoperative diagnosis is cancer)?

Step 2: Intra-operative assessment

- Look around. Does the patient have any other pathology that might affect their post-operative treatment plan (example: during the surgery for colon cancer, look for signs of metastatic disease)?

Step 3: Post-operative care **(NAGDIR)**

- Nursing (e.g. vitals, activity, diet, drains, pain medications)
- Antibiotics
- GI prophylaxis
- Deep venous prophylaxis
- Intravenous fluids
- Re-assess, Re-assess, Re-assess

At the end of the chapter, we have provided you with a mock oral examination in which we demonstrate how to use these two mnemonics when evaluating a clinical scenario.

Success tips

1. **Prepare for the examination.** It doesn't matter what surgical textbook you read, just be sure to read one. Know the presentation and treatment of common surgical diseases.

2. **Practice, Practice, Practice.** Need we say more?

3. **Be and look professional.** Set the stage for success by paying careful attention to your appearance, manner, and behavior. Establish a professional presence that will help you form a connection with your examiner.

During the Examination

Mistake #133

Letting your anxiety overwhelm you

It is natural to be nervous or anxious before and during the oral examination. In fact, a little nervousness or anxiety can be a good thing, keeping you on your toes and improving your overall performance. However, some students develop such a high level of anxiety that it negatively impacts their performance. It is important that you take the steps necessary to handle your feelings of nervousness and anxiety so that they don't affect your ability to perform up to your potential. Here are some tips that will help you decrease your nervousness and anxiety level:

- Visualize success. Imagine yourself impressing the examiner with your answers.

- Take the proper amount of time to prepare for the examination. This will certainly increase your confidence level.

- Reach the examination site 30 minutes before your scheduled examination time. Avoid rushing.

- On the way to the examination, listen to some inspiring music to motivate you.

- Before you walk through the door of the examining room, take a few deep breaths slowly in and out.

- Remind yourself that the oral examination is just one part of the grading process. In fact, in most surgery rotations, the weight the oral examination carries in the determination of your overall grade is significantly less than clinical evaluations and the written examination.

Mistake **#134**

Not being aware of your own nonverbal communication

During the oral examination, you will communicate in two ways - verbally and nonverbally. So much focus is placed on what we say that we often don't consider the way in which we say it or the manner in which we conduct ourselves. Successful nonverbal communication includes adhering to the following rules:

- Standing and walking with erect posture and shoulders back. Sit straight up in the chair, avoiding a slouched posture.

- Shaking hands firmly.

- Maintaining a relaxed face, making sure to avoid furrowing your brow, tensing your jaw, or looking too stern.

- Maintaining good eye contact. Avoid looking away or down, which are signs that you lack confidence.

- Keeping your hand gestures to a minimum.

- Avoiding nervous or distracting habits such as tapping your foot, drumming finger on a desk or chair, fiddling with jewelry, or twirling your hair.

Do not simply assume that you will not display these behaviors during the oral examination. Most students are not aware of their nonverbal communication and how it may affect their overall performance. Often, these tendencies come to light during a mock oral examination when your selected proctor points out not just what you are saying but also how you are saying it. In your practice sessions, be sure you ask your proctor about your nonverbal communication. If you learn that your nonverbal communication needs work, practice until you overcome the problem. By doing so, you will be able to portray a professional presence that will contribute to your overall success.

Mistake **#135**

Not listening to the question asked

There is a lot of information given at the beginning of an oral examination question. It is not a problem to take notes, but it is a problem to ask for data already verbalized. Consider the following example:

Examiner: A 54 year old female without past medical history presents with abdominal pain. What would you like to do?

Examinee: Does the patient have any significant past medical history?

This comment will be met with, "I said, no past medical history." This places you in an unpleasant situation, which could have been prevented by listening carefully to the question.

Mistake **#136**

Answering the question without thinking

All individuals are nervous when taking an oral examination. Therefore, it is critical to listen to the question and then mentally organize the answer into a logical sequence of events. Points are not taken off for a *short* pause to think; however, an improper or scattered answer will always be greeted with the perception that you are an disorganized individual, which will definitely lower your examination grade.

Mistake **#137**

Answering a question with a question

This is viewed as a stall tactic. Do not repeat any part of the question in your answer. If you didn't hear the question, ask for the question to be repeated. This will not hurt you, but excessive use will annoy the proctor and lower your score.

Mistake **#138**

Speaking inappropriately

Jargon and abbreviations are used every day while practicing medicine. However, during a formal examination, proper descriptions of procedures or tests should be verbalized. For example, a patient needs an abdominal perineal resection, not an APR. Proper communication allows the proctor to know that you are aware of the true procedure. The examinee should also avoid the use of proper names for procedures. For example a patient needs a pancreaticoduodenectomy for their pancreatic cancer not a Whipple.

Mistake #139

Answering a question when you truly don't know the answer

If you don't know the answer to a question, simply state, "I don't know." This will not lower your examination score; the proctor will probably re-phrase or choose an alternative question. You may be even given a hint or coaxed in some way that allows you to come up with the answer. Nevertheless, an "I don't know" answer should be limited to *once*. Sometimes, a question that is asked is not a student level question, which the proctor may be fully aware of. It is up to you to know your limitations and answer only those questions you feel that you can answer reasonably well.

Mistake #140

Thinking you can "read" the proctor

It's not unusual for proctors to try to get you to change your answer. In doing so they are testing your confidence. When you feel that a proctor is casting doubt about your decision plan, don't panic and more importantly do not change your answer. Most of the time you are correct, so "stick to your guns." Finally, a proctor will seldom reveal how you performed on a specific question. A proctor commonly continues the questioning to see what you actually know, or stops the questioning abruptly. Consider this behavior positive, not negative. Don't over analyze, and don't let this situation alter your confidence or affect the next question.

Success tips

Remember what your mother always taught you:

1. Sit up straight

2. Be polite

3. Pay attention

4. Think before you speak

5. Think positively

Mock oral examination

Examiner: 56-year old male presents to the emergency room with chief complaint of nausea, vomiting, and abdominal distention for 2 days prior to admission. He states he has not passed gas or had a bowel movement for two days. His past surgical history is significant for an appendectomy ten years ago and a past medical history for insulin dependent diabetes mellitus.

> Do not forget to begin with an assessment of the patient's ABCs (remember the "A" in the mnemonic AIDE stands for "assess ABC."

Student: I would like to perform my ABCs. Is the patient able to converse with me?

Examiner: Yes, and there are no signs of respiratory distress. However, the patient does complain of thirst.

Student: Well, the airway and breathing appear adequate. I would also like to know the patient's pulse and blood pressure.

Examiner: Heart rate is 110 and the initial blood pressure is 100/60.

Student: I'm concerned about his circulation. Since he is tachycardic and hypotensive, I would like to place two large bore intravenous catheters, bolus the patient with 2 liters of normal saline, and insert a Foley catheter. How is his heart rate and blood pressure after the fluid bolus?

Examiner: Heart rate is 90, with a blood pressure of 119/68.

After assessing the ABCs, offer your examiner your thoughts about what might be causing the patient's symptoms. (Remember the "I" in the mnemonic AIDE stands for "Institute differential diagnosis.")

Student: I'm concerned that the patient may have a bowel obstruction secondary to adhesions, hernia, or obstructing mass, or the patient may have acute pancreatitis, acute cholecystitis, gastroenteritis, perforated peptic ulcer, diverticulitis, or diabetic ketoacidosis.

Once you have provided the examiner with your differential diagnosis, you will need more information from the history and physical examination to determine which of the conditions in the differential diagnosis is the cause of the patient's clinical presentation. (Remember the "D" in the mnemonic AIDE stands for "determine pertinent positives and negative from the history and physical examination.") The examiner will assess your ability to collect relevant information from the history and physical examination.

Student: I need more information regarding his history and physical examination.

Examiner: What would you like to know?

Student: I would like to perform a physical examination. Could you tell me about his abdominal examination? Specifically, does the patient have peritonitis?

Examiner: No.

Student: On inspection does the patient appear distended? Are there any signs of bruising or erythema? Is there a visible hernia (i.e., inguinal, umbilical, incisional)?

Examiner: The abdomen is distended with a well-healed right lower quadrant incision. No hernias are noted.

Student: What are the qualities of the bowel sounds?

Examiner: Hyperactive and high-pitched.

Student: When I palpate the abdomen what do I find?

Examiner: The patient is tympanic with mild diffuse abdominal discomfort.

Student: On rectal examination, what do I find?

Examiner: Minimal stool in the vault, hemoccult negative, no masses.

> After asking the examiner questions to learn more about the patient's history and physical examination, you should have a better idea of the condition that is causing the patient's symptoms. At this point, you will want to let the examiner know about tests (e.g., laboratory, imaging, other) you would like to order to confirm the diagnosis, exclude other conditions in the differential diagnosis, and assess the severity of the illness. (Remember the "E" in the mnemonic AIDE stands for "establish appropriate tests to be ordered.") Your examiner will be assessing the appropriateness of the tests you would like to obtain.

Student: I would like to obtain serum electrolytes and complete blood count. I would also like to send the patient for an upright chest x-ray as well as flat and upright abdominal films.

Examiner: Laboratory results: WBC 12 K, H/H 14/47, platelets 400 K, Na 142, K 3.0, Cl 97, HCO_3 28, BUN 68, Creatinine 2.9, Serum Glucose 170.

Imaging results: Chest x-ray - normal, Flat and upright of abdomen - distended loops of bowel with multiple air fluid levels. No free air.

Student: Is there air in the rectum?

Examiner: Yes.

> Once you have received the information needed to make a diagnosis, state the diagnosis confidently along with your initial management plan.

Student: Sounds like a partial small bowel obstruction with evidence of dehydration and altered glucose metabolism. Since the patient does not demonstrate peritonitis or a complete obstruction, I would like to admit the patient, resuscitate with normal saline, replace potassium, and treat conservatively with a nasogastric tube, bowel rest, and serial abdominal exams.

Examiner: 24 hours later, the patient feels worse, had an episode of hemodynamic instability, and, on clinical examination, the patient has signs of peritonitis. Electrolytes are corrected and he is making 40 cc of urine per hour. What would you like to do?

Student: The patient needs an exploratory laparotomy. Since the patient is adequately volume resuscitated with normal electrolytes and has no comorbidities, I would like to proceed urgently to the operating room.

> Note that in the previous statement, the student has recognized that the patient's condition has changed and because of the change, surgery, rather than conservative therapy, is now warranted. When you decide that surgery is an appropriate course of action, you will want to use the mnemonic PIP, which stands for **p**reoperative, **i**ntraoperative, and **p**ostoperative assessment.

Examiner: You perform a midline exploration of the abdomen and find a single adhesive band wrapped around a segment of necrotic bowel with perforation and minimal contamination within the peritoneal cavity.

> When your examiner provides you with the findings of the operation, remember the "I" in PIP, which stands for intraoperative assessment. In other words, look around and ask yourself if the patient has any other pathology that might affect their intraoperative or postoperative treatment plan. (For example, during surgery for colon cancer, look for signs of metastatic disease).

Student: I would like to lyse the adhesion, perform a segmental small bowel resection to viable margins, and run the entire length of bowel from ligament of Treitz to the ileocecal valve. I would also examine the colon. If I do not see any other pathology within the abdomen, then I would perform a functional end-to-end anastomosis and close the fascia. But I would leave the skin open to heal via secondary intention.

Examiner: Okay, what do you want to do postoperatively?

> The last "P" in PIP stands for **p**ostoperative assessment. At this point, use the mnemonic NAGDIR to make sure you address the major aspects of postoperative care. NAGDIR = **n**ursing (e.g., vital signs, activity, diet, drains, pain medications), **a**ntibiotics, **G**I prophylaxis, **d**eep venous thrombosis prophylaxis, **i**ntravenous fluids, **r**e-assess the patient).

Student: I would like to admit the patient to the floor, monitor his vital signs, fluid status, and electrolytes closely, maintain the nasogastric tube until bowel function returns, and administer DVT prophylaxis until the patient is ambulating.

Examiner: On postoperative day #6, the patient develops acute onset of tachypnea and tachycardia.

Student: I am concerned about a pulmonary embolism, I want to obtain a pulmonary angiogram.

> Be familiar with the diagnosis and treatment of potential postoperative complications, including pulmonary embolism, myocardial infarction, wound infection, etc.

Examiner: Excellent. Let us proceed to the next question.

Studying for the Written Examination

Like other rotations, the surgery clerkship at most schools ends with a written examination. In the past, the faculty at each school was responsible for creating the clerkship examination. In recent years, however, an increasing number of schools have adopted the National Board of Medical Examiners (NBME) surgery examination as their end of clerkship test.

Students consider this examination to be challenging. The large volume of material that needs to be mastered, the demanding pace of the rotation, and long hours reduce the amount of time available for reading and studying.

So, while you are undoubtedly a very good test taker, the surgery clerkship will pose to you challenges that you may not have encountered in other rotations. In this chapter, we offer you practical and specific strategies that will help you not only adequately prepare for the examination but also maximize your examination performance.

Before the examination

Mistake **#141**

Underestimating the importance of the written examination

The weight the written examination score carries in the determination of the overall surgery rotation grade varies from one medical school to another. While evaluations of your clinical performance are generally more important than your written examination score, be sure you understand your clerkship's grading policy. Here are some important points to remember:

- A superb performance on the written examination will generally not make up for a poor performance on the wards.

- If you fail the examination, you will generally have to retake the examination or even repeat the entire clerkship, regardless of how stellar your clinical evaluations are.

- A passing examination score may not be sufficient to achieve honors, even if you have secured outstanding clinical evaluations. In some surgery rotations, you must exceed a certain score or percentile to be considered for an overall clerkship grade of honors.

Mistake **#142**

Not preparing for the examination using the right resources

While comprehensive textbooks of surgery are valuable resources, because of their length and level of detail, these books are not ideal for written examination preparation. A better approach is to use these books for patient-directed reading and to rely on shorter books for examination preparation. Opinions vary considerably among students regarding "the book" you should use but popular titles include *NMS Surgery, Essentials of General Surgery, Surgical Recall, High-Yield Surgery,* and *Blueprints in Surgery.* There seems to be much less debate about the importance of doing practice questions. Two popular sources of questions include *Surgery: PreTest Self-Assessment and Review* and *Appleton and Lange Review of Surgery.*

Mistake **#143**

Delaying examination preparation

Studying for the shelf examination should begin on Day #1 of the rotation. While surgery rotations may be two to three months in duration, days start early and end late, leaving students without considerable time to study.

The material that needs to be covered is large, and given the limits on your time, it is important to begin studying early in the rotation. An early start is the key to not only getting through the material but also in providing you with the time needed to properly review the subject matter before the examination.

Savvy students create a schedule to help them stay on track. This schedule should certainly be a reasonable one. It should not force you to do too much on a daily basis but yet allow you to cover all topics before the examination. If a busy day prevents you from reading about your scheduled topic, your schedule should afford you enough flexibility to catch up on a subsequent day.

Mistake #144

Letting your clinical performance slide as the examination nears

As the date of the shelf examination nears, students usually spend more time studying for the examination. While this is only natural, we caution you not to let your clinical performance slide. In the few hours that you have every evening, it is easy to spend the entire time studying for the examination. Do not forget that you have clinical responsibilities as well and your lack of attention to these duties (e.g., not preparing for the surgical case you will be scrubbing in on) as the examination nears has the potential to significantly hurt your clinical evaluation. Remember that an outstanding test score generally won't make up for a poor clinical evaluation.

Mistake **#145**

Reading only about general surgery

While some rotations expose their students to all branches of surgery, other clerkships may consist entirely or mainly of time spent on the general surgery service. In other words, students may not have the opportunity to take part in the care of patients on surgery subspecialty services such as orthopedic surgery, trauma surgery, and vascular surgery. If you find yourself in this situation, do not neglect the subject matter of these other subspecialties. Remember that the shelf examination will test you not only on your knowledge of general surgery but also the subspecialties of surgery.

We recommend that you take the time to review the content of the surgery shelf examination, which is provided in the following table. From this data taken from the National Board of Medical Examiners (NBME), you will see that a significant percentage of questions will come from the surgical subspecialties.

Content of the NBME surgery subject examination	
General principles	1-5%
Organ systems	
Immunologic disorders	1-5%
Diseases of the blood and blood-forming organs	5-10%
Diseases of the Nervous System and Special Senses	5-10%

Cardiovascular disorders	10-15%
Diseases of the Respiratory System	10-15%
Nutritional and digestive disorders	25-30%
Gynecologic disorders	5-10%
Renal, urinary, and male reproductive system	5-10%
Disorders of pregnancy, childbirth, and the puerperium	1-5%
Disorders of the skin and subcutaneous tissues	1-5%
Diseases of the musculoskeletal and connective tissue	5-10%
Endocrine and metabolic disorders	5-10%
Physician tasks	
Promoting health and health maintenance	1-5%
Understanding mechanisms of disease	20-25%
Establishing a diagnosis	45-50%
Applying principles of management	25-30%
From www.nbme.org	

Mistake #146

Not developing a reading plan or schedule

With the workday being so long, it can be difficult to find the time to read and study. With the relatively little reading time that you have, it is of obvious importance that you spend this time wisely, efficiently, and effectively. In the following, we offer you some reading tips.

Tips on reading and studying during the surgery clerkship

1. Determine the core information or material you need to be familiar with by the end of the rotation. You can obtain this information from your course syllabus, the NBME website (www.nbme.org), and your shelf examination review book.

2. Choose a book to use for examination preparation. Avoid the larger, more comprehensive texts, which will be difficult to get through in a two or three month rotation.

3. Develop a reading schedule or plan. If this plan is created properly and you are able to stay with the schedule, then you will avoid an all-too-common scenario—cramming just before the examination.

4. One recommended approach is to read the material you will be tested on twice, aiming to complete your reading two weeks before the examination. During the last two weeks, you can do your final review. For example, if your review book is 400 pages long, then you will need to read 11 pages a day to get through it twice by two weeks before the examination (assuming that your clerkship is 90 days in duration).

5. Consult your schedule every morning so that you know what you are expected to read for that particular day.

6. Take advantage of downtime during the day. You never know when time may present itself, in which case you will be prepared to use it to your advantage. Use the minutes that you find here and there to read. At the end of the day, you will be surprised what these

short blocks of time add up to. Many students are able to complete their scheduled reading during the workday while waiting for a lecture to begin, waiting for their surgical case to begin, or while on bus ride home, etc.

7. Carry copies of the chapters you are scheduled to read with you. It is often easier to carry copies of chapters than the book itself. Again, you never know when a short block of time may present itself. Be sure to have your reading materials handy.

8. Since reading about your patients' problems is one of the best ways you can prepare for the examination, read every evening about your patients' problems. For patient-directed reading, we recommend using one of the larger textbooks of surgery in addition to review books. If you are too tired, consider waking up a little bit earlier to read. Many people find that their concentration levels are higher early in the morning. Remember that it doesn't matter when you read but that you do read.

9. Since the focus of the examination is not on operative technique, do not spend too much time in this area. Instead, focus on anatomy, physiology, pathology, risk factors, symptoms, signs, differential diagnosis, testing (lab and radiologic abnormalities), treatment (surgical along with medical alternatives), prognosis, complications, and postoperative care of surgical problems.

10. Read actively. Don't forget that the surgery shelf examination, like other subject examinations developed by the NBME, "concentrate heavily on application and integration of knowledge rather than recall of isolated facts (from the subject examination program goals at www.nbme.org)." As you read about a problem, ask yourself if you would know how to establish the diagnosis and the treatment plan you

would recommend. Jot down notes, highlight, feed yourself questions, answer related practice questions, etc. Do whatever it takes to make sure that you have processed and understood the information.

11. If you fall behind, catch up on weekends. Unless you are on call, your responsibilities will generally be lighter.

During the examination

Mistake **#147**

Not pacing yourself

You are given two hours ten minutes to complete the 100-question surgery shelf examination or essentially a little over a minute per question. While this, at first, may seem like a reasonable amount of time, many students have had difficulty answering all questions in the time allotted.

What can you do to make sure you are able to finish the examination in the allotted time? First, realize that you have 1 minute 18 seconds per question. Since it isn't practical to time yourself as you read and answer every question, a better practice is to determine where you need to be at one quarter, one half, and three quarters of the time allotted to finish the examination.

Do not rely on the proctor to keep you abreast of the time —it is your own responsibility. You may or may not receive updates on how much time is remaining.

Success Tip #40

Do you find yourself easily disturbed by others when you take exams? If so, pick a part of the room that's less distracting for you. If noises bother you, consider wearing earplugs.

Success Tip #41

Do you often complete exams well before the allotted time has passed? Before you walk out the door, why not use the time that is left to make sure you coded responses on the answer sheet correctly? One of the authors of this book marked his answers in the wrong place, realizing his mistake just a minute or two before time was up.

Success Tip #42

You look up at the clock and you have two minutes remaining but you haven't read the last fifteen questions of the examination. What do you do? Pick a column and fill in the dots right down that column (i.e., fill in "C" for every item that is left). This approach is likely to yield more correct responses from a statistical standpoint.

Success Tip #43

If you finish the examination with time remaining, consider reviewing questions that gave you difficulty. Sometimes, something you read in one question might jog your memory or provide a clue to help you answer a previous question.

Success Tip #44

If you spend too much time on one question, it may cut down on the time you have to answer questions later. Don't miss easy questions located at the end of the examination because you spend too much time on question(s) at the beginning of the examination.

Mistake **#148**

Not reading the question first

The NBME states that questions on clinical science subject examinations, including the surgery shelf examination, are "framed in the context of clinical vignettes." These vignettes are often long and students have to read a considerable amount of information before they reach the question that is being asked. A better approach is to read the question first. In other words, instead of starting with the long clinical vignette that precedes the question, read the question first so that you know what to focus on in the vignette. After you read the question, be sure you understand it. As obvious as this may seem, this is one of the most common errors students make.

Mistake **#149**

Not reading each answer option

As you consider the answer choices, be sure that you read each option. Many students do not read each option, picking the first answer choice that seems like the best answer when, in fact, another option is the best and correct choice. Resist the temptation to select the first answer choice that seems right. Instead, consider each option carefully.

Mistake #150

Panicking

Anxiety can easily cause students to miss questions. Most students walk into the examination room feeling anxious, which, of course, is natural. A little bit of anxiety can certainly help your performance but too much anxiety can lead to test errors. Just before the examination, you must refrain from behaviors or conversations that might increase your anxiety level. Aim to arrive at the testing site 30 minutes before the examination begins. Some students, having arrived early, quiz each other right up until the examination starts. This is not likely to improve examination performance and, in fact, can have the opposite effect, especially if it significantly increases your anxiety level.

For many students, anxiety is more of a problem just after starting an examination. These students are prone to making errors early on the examination, mistakes that they are not likely to make once they regain their composure. If you recognize this tendency in yourself, set aside time at the end of the examination, if you can, to review your answers from the first ten or fifteen questions. You may pick up on errors. Another strategy to help you avoid these errors is to spend the ten or fifteen minutes before an examination answering practice questions. This strategy may help you focus and concentrate on the real test to come rather than on the anxiety you feel.

Success Tip #45

As you proceed through the examination, don't get caught up thinking about questions you have probably missed. You will feel your anxiety level rise, which will certainly affect your ability to focus on the question at hand. If you must worry about how many questions you may have missed, save it until after the examination ends.

101 Biggest Mistakes 3rd Year Medical Students Make and How to Avoid Them
ISBN # 0-9725561-0-9

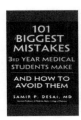

Compiled from discussions with hundreds of attending physicians, residents, and students, *101 Biggest Mistakes 3rd Year Medical Students Make And How To Avoid Them* discusses the major mistakes that students make during this very important year. Avoiding these pitfalls is the key to third-year success. This book will empower you, placing you in a position to have a successful experience, no matter what rotation or clerkship you are on. Once you are aware of these mistakes, you can do everything in your power to avoid them, thereby becoming the savvy student that is poised for clerkship success. Read what others have had to say:

"As someone who just matched into dermatology, I can tell you that residency program directors look closely at clerkship grades, especially for the more competitive residencies. *101 Biggest Mistakes 3rd Year Medical Students Make And How To Avoid Them* is a book that will help you get great clerkship grades."

—Review posted by Yang Xia on www.amazon.com

The Residency Match: 101 Biggest Mistakes and How to Avoid Them
ISBN # 0-9725561-1-7

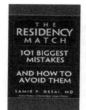

Are there any steps you can take to maximize your chances of matching with the residency program of your choice? One of the keys is to become familiar with the major mistakes that students make during the residency application process. These are mistakes that are well known to residency program directors but are not familiar to many applicants. In *The Residency Match: 101 Biggest Mistakes And How To Avoid Them*, we not only show you these mistakes but also help you avoid them, placing you in a position for match success. Read what others have had to say:

"The fourth year of medical school can be a stressful, demanding time. This book cuts down on the amount of necessary reading that you must do in order to match well. It has tips about subjects I had not thought about (for example, you should have a case ready to present your interviewer), as well as questions you will be asked in interviews and questions you should ask the interviewer. Overall, this is an easy to read book that I would definitely recommend because it contains all the essentials to matching in your ideal residency spot."

—Review posted by Jonathan Welch on www.amazon.com

Psychiatry Clerkship: 150 Biggest Mistakes and How to Avoid Them
ISBN # 0-9725561-5-X

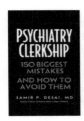

Many medical students find the psychiatry clerkship formidable, not because of a lack of knowledge about psychiatry, but because of a lack of preparation for actually doing the rotation. This "insider's guide" can help you shave weeks off the learning curve by identifying the most common and deleterious mistakes that medical students make, as well as the best approaches to avoiding them. Plus, the "must know" information contained in the appendices will be an invaluable resource in answering questions during rounds and preparing for your exam.

"A student who reads this prior to starting the psychiatry clerkship will be primed for an excellent experience."

—Timothy K. Wolff, M.D., Psychiatry Clerkship Coordinator
and Associate Professor of Psychiatry
University of Texas Southwestern Medical School

"This is a very useful and straightforward book that will successfully guide medical students through not only the psychiatry rotation, but many other clerkships as well."

—Anita Afzali, third year medical student
University of Washington School of Medicine

"The authors provide an astonishing amount of practical wisdom in easily understandable and readable prose. It deserves a place alongside the Washington manual in the pocket of every white coat in the halls of every medical school."

—Glenn O. Gabbard, M.D.,
Brown Foundation Chair of Psychoanalysis
Professor of Psychiatry, Baylor College of Medicine

Internal Medicine Clerkship: 150 Biggest Mistakes and How to Avoid Them
ISBN # 0-9725561-2-5

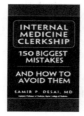

Did you know that most medical students begin doing their best work at the end of the Internal Medicine clerkship? Wouldn't it be great if there were a book available that could speed up the learning curve so that students were performing at a high level right from the get-go? Now with the *Internal Medicine Clerkship: 150 Biggest Mistakes And How To Avoid Them*, there's absolutely no reason to save your best for last. Read what others have had to say:

"I read the book cover to cover prior to starting the rotation, and it helped me get off to a great start. I feel the book had a great influence on both my performance as a clinical student and my evaluation by my teammates. Overall, an extremely helpful and eye opening text. I attribute much of my success to the wisdom I gathered from this book."

—Brian Broaddus, after completing his Internal Medicine clerkship at the Baylor College of Medicine

Pediatrics Clerkship: 101 Biggest Mistakes and How to Avoid Them
ISBN # 0-9725561-4-1

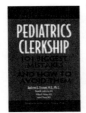

The Pediatrics Clerkship is different in several respects from every other core clerkship you will have in medicine, and many students are uncertain of how to successfully navigate the transition from adult care to the care of children. This book eases the transition by introducing students to the all-too-common mistakes that are made during the clerkship. Armed with this knowledge, students will be able to avoid these mistakes, which will increase their clerkship enjoyment, learning, and performance.

"This book should be titled *Success on the Wards*. It not only gives advice specific to a pediatrics clerkship, but the general do's and don'ts of any rotation. The lessons are clear, concise and will save any medical student both time and energy—not to mention the ability to impress attendings and residents."
—Samira L. Brown, 4th year Medical Student
Harvard Medical School

"This book is well worth the attention of every medical student who wants to optimize their time on his/her pediatrics clerkship. It covers all the bases on how a medical student should approach their clinical roles, responsibilities, and education during every aspect of the pediatric experience whether in the inpatient setting, the ambulatory setting, or the nursery. Reading this book will prepare the medical student to learn how to care for children of all ages, interact with parents and other care providers, and work most effectively within the pediatric team. There are wonderful suggestions throughout the book, including tips on how to perform a physical examination on even the most challenging toddler."

—Melanie S. Kim, M.D., Associate Professor,
Boston University School of Medicine,
Department of Pediatrics

Associate Director of Residency Training,
Boston Combined Residency Program in Pediatrics

Deputy Editor, *UpToDate in Pediatrics*
Editorial Board, *Contemporary Pediatrics*

MD2B Titles

101 Biggest Mistakes 3rd Year Medical Students Make and How to Avoid Them

The Residency Match: 101 Biggest Mistakes and How to Avoid Them

Internal Medicine Clerkship: 150 Biggest Mistakes and How to Avoid Them

Surgery Clerkship: 150 Biggest Mistakes and How to Avoid Them

Pediatrics Clerkship: 101 Biggest Mistakes and How to Avoid Them

Psychiatry Clerkship: 150 Biggest Mistakes and How to Avoid Them

View sample chapters of these books at www.md2b.net

About www.md2b.net

Our website, www.md2b.net, is committed to helping today's medical student become tomorrow's doctor. The site is dedicated to providing students with the tools needed to tackle the challenges of medical school. The website provides the following information:

Survival Guides for 3rd Year Clerkships
Success tips (tips of the week)
Introduction to the residency match
Residency Match tips

—AND MUCH MORE!